A Textbook on Food, Nutrition and Dietetics

by
Dr. Debasish Kundu
M.D.H., F.F.Hom, F.I.H.M.S., Ph.D. (U.S.A.), D.Sc. (Colombo)

Editor
Dr. Malik A.K. Awan
B.S., M.S. (Psychology), M.D. (A.M.), D.C.L., D.D. (U.S.A.), Ph.D. (London)

Associate Editor
Prof. Seyed Farzin Hassanzadeh Salehian
M.D., Diploma TCM, Ph.D., D.Sc.

ORIGINALS

Originals
Delhi

First Published 2018

ISBN 10: 81-8454-187-2
ISBN 13: 978-81-8454-187-8

Published by
Originals
(an imprint of Low Price Publications)
A-6, 2nd Floor, Nimri Commercial Centre,
Ashok Vihar Phase 4, Delhi 110052 (INDIA)
tel.: +91-11-27302453 fax.: +91-11-47061936
url: www.LPPindia.com e-mail: info@LPPindia.com

Printed at
Monica Enterprises
Delhi

PRINTED IN INDIA

Contents

Preface

The primary objective of nutrition and diet is to address the nutritional qualities of a food factually and informatively, thereby assisting the consumer in making better food choices when planning their daily meals.

The book been designed keeping in view of the need of nutritionists, dieticians, medical doctors and food scientists.

It is hoped that this book will be able to assist the food industry, the regulatory authorities, all related professionals and the consumers in the understanding and application of the nutrition and diet for human health.

Dr. Debasish Kundu
drdkundu@msn.com

1

Relationship between Food, Nutrition & Health

Food has been a basic part of our existence. By knowing the food composition, the nutritional content of food is known.

Intake of food ensures growth in children and youth, maintains good health throughout life, meets special needs of pregnancy and lactation and for recovery from illness.

A large part of our food heritage is scientifically beneficial and needs to be retained, some aspects may need to be modified in view of changes in our lifestyles.

Most of the articles are published in papers and journals may be correct but most of it may not be.

Therefore this course will give a proper information on food and the knowledge gained can be spread to people around, so that the false ideas about foods which interfere with food selection are erased and health is not affected

Definitions

Food–is one that nourishes the body.

Food may also be defined as any substance eaten or drunk which meets the needs for energy, body building, regulation and protection of the body.

Food is the material from which our bodies are made.

Eating right kind of food in right amounts ensures good nutrition and health.

Nutrition–is food at work in the body. It includes everything that happens from eating food to its usage in various functions of body.

Nutrients are components of foods needed for body in adequate amounts for proper growth, reproduction and leading normal life.

The science of nutrition deals with what nutrients we need, in what quantity, how to get them and how the body utilizes them.

Adequate, optimum and good nutrition – indicates the right amount and proportion of nutrients for proper utilization for achieving highest level of physical and mental health.

Nutritional status – state of the body as a result of foods consumed and their utilization by the body. Nutritional status can be good, fair and poor.

Good nutritional status–characterized by an alert, good natured personality, a well developed body with normal weight for height, well developed and firm muscles, healthy skin, reddish pink coloured eyelids and membranes of mouth, good layer of subcutaneous fat, clear eyes, smooth and glossy hair, good appetite and excellent general health which is recognized by stamina to work, regular meal time, sound sleep, normal elimination and resistance to disease.

Health–as defined by WHO is the 'state of complete physical, mental and social well being and not mere absence of disease or infirmity'.

Malnutrition–undesirable kind of nutrition leading to ill health. It results from lack, excess or imbalance of nutrients in the diet. It includes both under and over nutrition. Under nutrition is a state of insufficient supply of essential nutrients.

Malnutrition can be primarily due to insufficient supply of one or more essential nutrients or it can be secondary, which means it results from an error in metabolism, interaction between nutrients or nutrients and drugs used for treatment.

Over nutrition refers to an excessive intake of one or more nutrients which creates a stress on bodily functions.

Diet–refers to whatever is eaten or drunk each day. It includes normal diet that is consumed either individually or in groups. Diets may be modified for making it suitable for sick individuals as a part of treatment – therapeutic diets

Nutritional care–using knowledge of nutrition for meal planning and preparation to make it in an attractive and acceptable form. In this the existing meals can be modified to improve in terms of nutrition, and acceptability. Diet can be planned for individuals or a group to suit their requirements like health status, nutritional status, place of living, climate etc.

Functions of food

Physiological functions of food

First function of food is to provide energy. Body needs energy to sustain involuntary processes essential for continuing life. It is also required for various activities like professional, household and recreational activities, convert foods into utilizable nutrients required for growth and warmth.

Another important function is body building. An infant at birth weighs 2.5-3.0 kgs. and grows to 50-60 kgs. during adulthood, which is possible only if right food in right amount is given from birth to adulthood. Food eaten also help to maintain the structure of the body and helps in repair of worn out tissues.

Food regulates the activities of the body including – heart beat, maintaining body temperature, muscle contraction, water balance, blood clotting and removal of waste products from the body.

Food helps in improving the immune system and improves resistance power of the body.

Social functions of food

Food has always been the central part of our existence, social cultural and religious life.

Special foods are distributed during religious functions in homes, temples, churches etc.

Feasts are given in different stages of life like birth, cradle ceremony, birthdays, marriages etc. many feasts call for feeding specific segment of people.

Certain menus are associated with specific foods in each region.

Food has been used as expression of love friendship and social acceptance.

Food is also used to express happiness like success in exams, job, marriages, birth of a baby etc.

Food for get together, meetings or functions should be planned in a proper manner to bring people together.

Psychological functions of food

In addition to physical and social needs, food must satisfy certain emotional needs.

It includes a sense of security, love and attention.

Familiar foods usually make us feel secure.

Sharing of food is a token of friendship and acceptance.

In a friendly gathering we try unfamiliar foods and thus enlarge our food experiences.

Anticipating needs and fulfilling these are expressions of love and attention.

These sentiments are the basis of the normal attachment to mother's cooking or home food.

If the foods included are unfamiliar or not tasty, then even nutritionally balanced foods may not be satisfactory.

With time and repeated experience unfamiliar and strange foods become familiar and one develops taste for those foods.

Therefore these aspects are to be kept in mind while planning meals which are nutritionally adequate and also enjoyable.

2
History of Nutrition

Man has always been concerned about food, along with the two other factors basic to living, namely, shelter and clothing. He apparently began his life as a carnivorous animal, he was a hunter of game and a fisherman. Only at the end of the Stone Age he did begin to cultivate grains for food and add berries and honey to his staple, meat.

Archaeological evidence reveals that the development of communities, towns and cities came through the setting of groups of people to cultivate foods. Men of ancient times offered theories about the health values of specific foods. Some of their wisdom is recorded in historical, philosophical treatises and in chapters in the Bible.

During the eighteenth century when scientific discoveries were changing concepts and causing intellectual ferment, the French chemist Antoine Laurent Lavoisier recognized the relationship of the process of respiration to the metabolism of food. He had discovered the role of oxygen and combustion and investigated the relationship of the burning flame to the metabolism of organic foods. Lavoisier is called the father of nutrition.

In 1896 W.O. Atwater, who has been called "the father of American nutrition", published the first extensive table of food values ever published in this country. At that time, only proteins and calories were generally considered to be of nutritional importance. It was not until 20 years later that E.V. McCollum one of the principal early workers in the field of accessory food factors, popularized the concept of "protective foods" those primarily used for their content of vitamins and minerals. Shortly after W.W. 1 this resulted in a marked increase in the consumption of leafy vegetables, citrus fruit and milk.

At the same time, Graham Lusk was experimenting his far-reaching influence on dietary habits. As expert on calorie needs, it was he who first secured popular acceptance of the fact that adolescents require as much food as adults.

An abundance of reading material is available for exploration by the interested student.

Importance of Food

Food is the prime necessary factor sustaining life. The religious book "Geeta" recognises the basic dictum of food for warm blooded animals, to maintain the specific body temperature, which differs from a dead body. A living thing requires a continuous supply of heat and energy which is provided by the slow oxidation of food. This energy is transformed into kinetic energy to form various activities of the body like grinding of teeth, working of brain, heart functioning, muscular movements etc., The body is able to regulate the heat better. The burning of carbon is not direct. It is simplified into various intermediates substances. CO_2 and water are the end products.

The metabolic path way is called 'Kreb's Cycle' The heat produced during oxidation of glucose and other carbon compound, is trapped in the form of chemical energy by the formation of compounds with high energy phosphate. The tissues formed are also constantly being renewed without loss of continuity in structure and function. This is possible because they are constantly being renewed without loss of continuity in structure and function. This is possible because they are constantly broken down to their constituents and resynthesised. In carder to maintain warm temperature, the body must not only build itself but also repair the damaged tissues. The building or each tissue proceeds in a different way.

The Brain contains large amount of Lipids, Bones, minerals, The body functions because of nutrients present in food and of the capacity of body to utilise them. The nutrients needed by the body are proteins, Fats, Carbohydrates, Vitamins, minerals and water, Certain food, Vegetables and oil contain exclusively fat and other food such as sugars, exclusively CHO. But most common food have several nutrients in varying proportions. The chief compounds utilised in the body during heat production are CHO, proteins, and fat. Oxidation takes place by a series of slow reactions which requires enzymes. Enzymes are biological catalysts which make it possible for the chemical reaction to occur at body temperature. Most of them require specific Vitamins, minerals, water, protein and fat for then specific activities. Although carbohydrate is the major source of fuel, it is limited and they require it either by food or from the body's store of fat and proteins. The body also contains substantial quantity of calcium, inorganic salts and other Vitamins. In general, health, physical appearances and performances of work depends on the quantity and adequacy of the food intake.

Every culture has its dietary patterns based the uses of various food such as cereals, legumes, Vegetables fruits, nuts, milk, meat, fish, egg. In some culture the use of non vegetarian is taboo (Prohibited).

E.g.: Eskimos, hunting tribes, primitive man have instinctively formed adequate dietary habits by survives, for many years. But as a result of modern food technology and urbanization food patterns have changed.

These changes have affected the health of modern man

E.g.: Introduction chillies, Coffee, Tea and highly milled rice etc.

3
Functions of Food

Body Composition & the Functions of Food

The phrase "we are what we eat" is frequently used to signify that the composition of our bodies is dependent in large measure on what we have consumed.

The many chemical elements in the human body occur mainly in the form of water, protein, fats, mineral salts and carbohydrates during bodily processes. Each human body is built up from food containing these five constituents, and vitamins as well.

Food serves mainly for growth, energy and body repair, maintenance and protection. Food also provides enjoyment and stimulation, since eating and drinking are among the pleasures of life everywhere. Truly food nourishes both the body and soul. Even if technology could produce a perfect diet in terms of content, such a diet could still lack, for example, the aroma and flavour of a curry, or the stimulating taste of hot coffee.

What controls appetite or the feeling of hunger is not fully understood. The hypothalamus in the brain has a role, as do other central nervous system sites. Other probable factors include blood sugar levels, body hormones, body fat, many diseases, emotions and of course food type and availability, personal likes and dislikes and the social setting where food is to be consumed.

Dietary Constituents and the Functions of Food

Human beings eat food, and not individual nutrients. Most foods, including staples such as rice, maize and wheat, provide mainly carbohydrate for energy but also significant quantities of protein, a little fat or oil and useful micronutrients. Thus cereal grains provide some of the constituents needed for energy, growth and body repair and maintenance. Breastmilk provides all the macro and micronutrients necessary to satisfy the total needs of a young infant up to six months of age including those for energy, growth and body repair and maintenance. Cows' milk has the balance of nutrients for all the requirements of a calf.

Functions of Water

Water can be considered the most important dietary constituent. A normal man or woman can live without food for 20 to 40 days, but without water humans die in four to seven days. Over 60 per cent of human body weight is made up of water, of which approximately 61 per cent is intracellular and the rest extracellular. Water intake, except under exceptional circumstances (e.g. intravenous feeding), comes from the food and fluids consumed. The amount consumed varies widely in individuals and may be influenced by climate, culture and other factors. Often as much as 1 litre is consumed in solid food, and 1 to 3 litres as fluids drunk. Water is also formed in the body as a result of oxidation of macronutrients, but the water thus obtained usually constitutes less than 10 per cent of total water.

Water is excreted mainly by the kidneys as urine. The kidneys regulate the output of urine and maintain a balance;

if smaller amounts of fluid are consumed, the kidneys excrete less water, and the urine is more concentrated. While most water is eliminated by the kidneys, in hot climates as much or more can be lost from the skin (through perspiration) and the lungs. Much smaller quantities are lost from the gut in the faeces (except in the presence of diarrhoea, when losses may be high).

Table: Chemical Composition of a Human Body Weighing 65 kg

Component	Percentage of Body Weight
Water	61.6
Protein	17
Fats	13.8
Minerals	6.1
Carbohydrate	1.5

Table: Simple Classification of Dietary Constituents

Constituent	Use
Water	To provide body fluid and to help regulate body temperature
Carbohydrates	As fuel for energy for body heat and work
Fats	As fuel for energy and essential fatty acids
Proteins	For growth and repair
Minerals	For developing body tissues and for metabolic processes and protection
Vitamins	For metabolic processes and protection
Indigestible and Unabsorbable Particles, including Fibre	To form a vehicle for other nutrients, add bulk to the diet, provide a habitat for bacterial flora and assist proper elimination of refuse

Metabolism of sodium and potassium, which are known as electrolytes, is linked with body water. The sodium is mainly in the extracellular water and the potassium in the intracellular water. Most diets contain adequate amounts of both these minerals. In fluid loss caused, for example, by diarrhoea or haemorrhage, the balance of electrolytes in the blood may become disturbed. Water intake and electrolyte balance are particularly important in sick infants. In healthy infants, breastmilk alone from a healthy mother provides adequate quantities of fluids and electrolytes without additional water for the first six months of life even in hot climates. Infants with diarrhoea and disease, however, may require additional fluids.

While food intake is largely regulated by appetite and food availability, fluid intake is influenced by the sensation termed thirst. Thirst may arise for various reasons. In dehydration it may be caused by drying of the mouth but also by signals from the same satiety centre in the hypothalamus that controls hunger sensations. Dehydration, an important feature of diarrhoea.

The phenomenon of water accumulation in the body is manifested in the condition known as oedema, when disease causes an excess of extracellular fluid. Two important deficiencydiseases in which generalized oedema is a feature are kwashiorkor and wet beriberi. The excess fluid may result from electrolyte disturbances and accumulation of water in the extracellular compartment. A person can have oedema and still be dehydrated from diarrhoea; this condition is a form of heart failure. Water can also collect in the peritoneal cavity, in the condition known as ascites, which may be caused by liver disease.

Composition of Human Body

The human body is sometimes said to be divided into three compartments, accounting for the following shares of the total body weight of a well-nourished healthy adult male:

Body cell mass, 55 per cent.
Extracellular supporting tissue, 30 per cent.
Body fat, 15 per cent.

The body cell mass is made up of cellular components such as muscle, body organs (viscera, liver, brain, etc.) and blood. It comprises the parts of the body that are involved in body metabolism, body functioning, body work and so on.

The extracellular supporting tissue consists of two parts: the extracellular fluid (for example, the blood plasma supporting the blood cells) and the skeleton and other supporting structures.

Body fat is nearly all present beneath the skin (subcutaneous fat) and around body organs such as the intestine and heart. It serves in part as an energy reserve. Small quantities are present in the walls of body cells or in nerves.

Physiologists and those interested in metabolism have developed various ways to estimate body composition, including the amount of fluids in the body and body density. A common determination is to estimate lean body mass (LBM) or the fat-free mass of the body. These measures vary from the very simple to the very difficult. The simpler ones are of course less precise. Anthropometry using weight, height, skinfold thickness and body circumferences is relatively easy and very cheap to undertake, and does provide some estimate of LBM and body composition. In contrast, methods using, for example, bioelectrical impedance, computerized axial tomography (CAT scans) and nuclear magnetic resonance require expensive apparatus and highly trained staff.

The fluid in the cells (intracellular fluid) has mainly potassium ions, and the extracellular fluid is mainly a solution of sodium chloride. Both also have other ions. Total body water can be estimated using different methods including dilution techniques to measure, for example, plasma volume.

Body fat is estimated using different methods. Because a large portion of adipose tissue is present beneath the skin, it can be estimated by using a skinfold calliper to measure skinfold thickness in different sites. Another method is to weigh the person both in air and under water using a special apparatus and tank. This method really provides an estimate of body density.

The various methods of determining body composition are described in detail in textbooks of physiology.

Body composition is much influenced by nutrition. The two extremes are the wasting of nutritional marasmus and starvation and the overweight of obesity. Body composition differs between the genders and, perhaps only slightly, among races. African Americans have been shown to have heavier skeletons than whites of the same body build in the United States. In females pregnancy and lactation influence body composition.

The body composition of children is influenced by their age and growth. Disturbances of growth resulting from nutritional deficiencies influence body composition, including the eventual size of the body and of body organs.

Metabolism and Energy

The general term for all the chemical processes carried out by the cells of the body is "metabolism". Chief among these processes is the oxidation (combustion, or burning) of food which produces energy. This process is analogous to a car engine burning petrol to produce the energy that makes it run. In most forms of combustion, be it in the car or in the human, heat is produced as well as energy.

Classical physics taught that energy can be neither created nor destroyed. Although this law of nature is not completely correct (as the conversion of matter to energy in a nuclear reactor shows), it is still true in most instances. All three macronutrients in food - carbohydrate, protein and fat provide energy. Energy for the body comes mainly from food, and in the absence of food it can be produced only by the breakdown of body tissues.

All forms of energy can be converted into heat energy. It is possible to measure the heat produced by burning a litre of petrol, for example. Food energy can also be and is expressed as heat energy. The unit of measurement used has been the large calorie (Cal) or kilocalorie (kcal) (which is 1 000 times the small calorie used in physics), but this measure is increasingly being replaced by the joule (J) or kilojoule (kJ). The kilocalorie is defined as the heat necessary to raise the temperature of 1 litre of water from 14.5° to 15.5°C. Whereas the kilocalorie is a unit of heat, the joule is truly a unit of energy. The joule is defined as the amount of energy used when 1 kg is moved 1 m by 1 newton (N) of force. In nutrition the kilojoule (1000 j) is used. The equivalent of 1 kcal is 4.184 kj. These are units of measurement in the same way that litres and pints are measures of quantity, and metres and feet are measures of length. In many scientific journals the joule is being introduced in place of the kilocalorie, but the general public and most health workers still prefer to express food energy in kilocalories rather than joules.

The human body requires energy for all bodily functions, including work, the maintenance of body temperature and the continuous action of the heart and lungs In children energy is essential for growth Energy is also needed for breakdown, repair and building of tissues. These arc metabolic processes.

The rate at which these functions are carried out while the body is at rest is the Basal metabolic rate (BMR).

Basal Metabolic Rate

BMR for an individual person is usually defined as the amount of energy [expressed in kilocalories or megajoules (MJ), per day] expended when the person is at complete rest, both physical (i.e. lying down) and psychological. It can also be expressed as kilocalories per hour or per kilogram of weight. BMR provides the energy required by the body for maintenance of body temperature; for the work of body organs such as the beating heart and the muscles working for normal, at rest, breathing; and for the functioning of other organs such as the liver, kidneys and brain.

BMR varies from individual to individual. Important general factors influencing BMR are the person's weight, gender, age and state of health. BMR is also influenced by the person's body composition, for example the amounts of muscle and adipose tissue and therefore the amounts of protein and fat in the body.

In broad terms, bigger people with more muscle and larger body organs have higher BMR than smaller people.

Elderly people tend to have lower BMR than they had when they were young, and females tend to have lower BMR than males even on a per kilogram body weight basis. There are exceptions, however, to all these generalizations.

BMR is important as a component of energy requirements. Table below shows BMR of adult men and women according to height and weight, both per kilogram body weight and as total energy per day.

The table shows, for example, that in females aged 30 to 60 years BMR ranges from 1,190 to 1,420 kcal per day.

This is the amount of energy required by a woman at complete rest for 2 hours. Of course many adult females in developing countries are smaller than 1.4 m in height and 41 kg in weight; their BMR might then be a little lower than 1,190 kcal per day.

Energy Requirements

The mean daily energy requirements of adult men and women doing work classified as light, moderate and heavy are given in table, expressed as multiples of BMR.

The table shows, for example, that a woman doing heavy work requires energy equal to 1.32 times her BMR. If the woman is aged 25 years, is 1.4 m tall and weighs 41 kg, according to Table her BMR would be 1100 kcal per day. Thus her daily requirements are: 1,100 kcal x 1.32 = 2,002 kcal.

It is often useful to estimate energy needs for various activities that a person may do for particular lengths of time.

The energy expenditure is usually calculated by multiplying an activity factor or metabolic constant, which varies according to the activity, by the individual's BMR.

Table gives the activity factors for calculating gross energy expenditure of various activities for adult males and females.

The average human burns energy at his or her BMR only when at complete rest. All ordinary movements require additional energy, and physical work, of course, requires more still. For a healthy male with BMR of 1 kcal/min, an average day may involve the energy expenditure shown in the below Tables.

Table: Average Daily Energy Requirements of Adults by Category of Occupational Work Expressed as a Multiple of BMR

Classification of Work	Men	Women
Light	1.55	1.56
Moderate	1.78	1.64
Heavy	2.10	1.82

Table: Activity Factors for Calculating Gross Energy Expenditure (Multiply by BMR)

Activity	Adult Males	Adult Females
Sleeping	1.0	1.0
Lying	1.2	1.2
Sitting quietly	1.2	1.2
Standing quietly	1.5	1.5
Walking slowly	2.8	2.8
Walking at normal pace	3.2	3.3
Walking fast uphill	7.5	6.6
Cooking	1.8	1.8
Office work (moving around)	1.6	1.7
Driving lorry	1.4	1.4
Labouring	5.2	4.4
Cutting sugar cane	6.5	
Pulling loaded cart	5.9	
Playing soccer	6.6	6.3
Fetching water from well		4.1
Pounding grain		4.6

Note: These values apply only as approximate mean values

for the time actually spent on the activity. They do not allow for rests. In heavy work individuals usually take frequent pauses or rests.

If the person in this example did instead of eight hours of light work - five hours of herding and three hours of heavy work, hoeing hard ground at 8 kcal/min., then his output of energy would be as shown in Table.

If the individual undertaking the activities in the first example gets exactly 2 640 kcal in his food, his weight will be steady, and he will be functioning normally.

However, if he then undertakes the activities in the second example and eats no extra food, his weight will gradually drop, because he will have to burn up his fuel reserve, which forms part of his own body. He would fairly soon, however, begin to limit his activities in order to stop this process.

He would therefore probably work much less hard at hoeing, so that instead of burning 8 kcal/min. he might use only, say, 3.2 kcal/min.: he would also tend to be tired at the end of the day, and might well increase his period of complete rest (at 1 kcal/min.) by reducing the period of minor activities. He would therefore have reduced his energy requirements to 2 646 kcal.

This is just an example. In most in stances, when people increase their output of energy, including work, they feel more hungry and increase their consumption of their staple food, be it rice, millet, maize wheat, cassava or anything else.

The energy requirements of human being are affected by several factors. The important ones are:

Body size: A small person needs less energy than a large person.

Basal metabolic rate: BMR varies and can be affected by factors such as disease of the thyroid gland.

Activity: The more physical work or recreation performed, the more energy is required.

Pregnancy: A woman requires extra energy to develop the foetus and to carry its additional weight.

Lactation: The lactating mother needs additional energy to produce energy-containing milk for the suckling baby. The relatively long duration of breastfeeding among most Asians and Africans results in a large proportion of women requiring extra energy.

Age: Infants and children need more energy, for growth and activity, than adults. In older persons, the need for energy is sometimes reduced because there is a decline in activity and because their BMR is usually lower.

Climate: In warm climates, i.e. in most of the tropics and subtropics, less energy is necessary to keep the body at its normal temperature than in cold climates.

Macronutrients: Carbohydrates, Fats and Proteins

Carbohydrates

The main source of energy for most Asians, Africans and Latin Americans is carbohydrates in the food they eat. Carbohydrates constitute by far the greatest portion of their diet, as much as 80 per cent in some cases. In contrast, carbohydrates make up only 45 to 50 per cent of the diet of many people in industrialized countries.

Carbohydrates are compounds containing carbon, hydrogen and oxygen in the proportions 6:12:6.

They are burned during metabolism to produce energy, liberating carbon dioxide (C02) and water (H20). The carbohydrates in the human diet are mainly in the form of starches and various sugars. Carbohydrates can be divided into three groups:

Monosaccharides, e.g. glucose, fructose, galactose;

Disaccharides, e.g. sucrose, lactose, maltose;

Polysaccharides, e.g. starch, glycogen (animal starch), cellulose.

Monosaccharides

The simplest carbohydrates are the monosaccharides, or simple sugars. These sugars can pass through the wall of the alimentary tract without being changed by the digestive enzymes. The three most common are glucose, fructose and galactose.

Glucose, sometimes also called dextrose, is present in fruit, sweet potatoes, onions and other plant substances. It is the substance into which many other carbohydrates, such as the disaccharides and starches, are converted by the digestive enzymes. Glucose is oxidized to produce energy, heat and carbon dioxide, which is exhaled in breathing.

Because glucose is the sugar in blood, it is most often used as an energy-producing substance for persons fed intravenously. Glucose dissolved in sterile water, usually in concentrations of 5 or 10 per cent, is frequently used for this purpose.

Fructose is present in honey and some fruit juices. Galactose is a monosaccharide that is formed, along with glucose, when the milk sugar lactose is broken down by the digestive enzymes.

Disaccharides

The disaccharides, composed of simple sugars, need to be converted by the body into monosaccharides before they can be absorbed from the alimentary tract.

Examples of disaccharides are sucrose, lactose and maltose. Sucrose is the scientific name for table sugar (the kind that is used, for example, to sweeten tea).

It is most commonly produced from sugar cane but is also produced from beets. Sucrose is also present in carrots and pineapple. Lactose is the disaccharide present in human and animal milk. It is much less sweet than sucrose. Maltose is found in germinating seeds.

Polysaccharides

The polysaccharides are chemically the most complicated carbohydrates. They tend to be insoluble in water, and only some can be used by human beings to produce energy. Examples of polysaccharides are starch, glycogen and cellulose.

Starch is an important source of energy for humans. It occurs in cereal grains as well as in root foods such as potatoes and cassava. Starch is liberated during cooking when the starch granules rupture because of heating.

Glycogen is made in the human body and is sometimes known as animal starch. It is formed from monosaccharides produced by the digestion of dietary starch. Starch from rice or cassava is broken down in the intestines to form monosaccharide molecules, which pass into the bloodstream. Those surplus monosaccharides that are not used to produce energy (and carbon dioxide and water) are fused together to form a new polysaccharide, glycogen. Glycogen is usually present in muscle and in the liver, but not in large amounts.

Any of the digestible carbohydrates when consumed in excess of body needs are converted by the body into fat which is laid down as adipose tissue beneath the skin and at other sites in the body.

Cellulose, hemicellulose, lignin, pectin and gums are sometimes called unavailable carbohydrates because humans cannot digest them. Cellulose and hemicellulose are plant polymers that are the main components of cell walls.

They are fibrous substances. Cellulose,which is a polymer of glucose, is one of the fibres of green plants. Hemicellulose is a polymer of other sugars, usually hexose and pentose. Lignin is the main component of wood.

Pectins are present in plant tissue and sap and are colloidal polysaccharides. Gums are also viscous carbohydrates extracted from plants. Pectins and gums are both used by the food industry. The human alimentary tract cannot break down these carbohydrates or utilize them to produce energy. Some animals, such as cattle, have microorganisms in their intestines that break down cellulose and make it available as an energy-producing food. In humans, any of the unavailable carbohydrates present in food pass through the intestinal tract. They form much of the bulk and roughage evacuated in human faeces, and are often termed as dietary fibre.

There is increasing interest in fibre in diets, because high-fibre diets are now considered healthful. A clear advantage of a high-fibre diet is a lower incidence of constipation than among people who consume a low-fibre diet. The bulk in high-fibre diets may contribute a feeling of fullness or satiety which may lead to less consumption of energy, and this may help reduce the likelihood of obesity. A high-fibre diet results in more rapid transit of food through the intestinal tract and is thus believed to assist normal and healthy intestinal and bowel functioning. Dietary fibre has also been found to bind bile in the intestines.

It is now recognized that the high fibre content of most traditional diets may be an important factor in the prevention of certain diseases which appear to be much more prevalent in people consuming the low-fibre diets common in industrialized countries. Because it facilitates the rapid passage of materials through the intestine, fibre may be a factor in the control of diverticulitis, appendicitis, haemorrhoids and also possibly arteriosclerosis, which leads to coronary heart disease and some cancers.

Frequent consumption of any sticky fermentable carbohydrates, either starch or sugar, can contribute to dental caries, particularly when coupled with poor oral hygiene. Adequate intake of fluoride and/or a topical application is the best protection against caries.

Fats

In many developing countries dietary fats make up a smaller part of total energy intake (often only 8 or 10 per cent) than carbohydrates. In most industrialized countries the proportion of fat intake is much higher. In the United States, for example, an average of 36 per cent of total energy is derived from fat.

Fats, like carbohydrates, contain carbon, hydrogen and oxygen. They are insoluble in water but soluble in such chemical solvents as ether, chloroform and benzene. The term 'fat' is used here to include all fats and oils that are edible and occur in human diets, ranging from those that are solid at cool room temperatures, such as butter, to those that are liquid at similar temperatures, such as groundnut or cottonseed oils.

Fats (also referred to as lipids) in the body are divided into two groups: storage fat and structural fat. Storage fat provides a reserve storehouse of fuel for the body, while the structural fats are part of the essential structure of the cells, occurring in cell membranes, mitochondria and intracellular organelles.

Cholesterol is a lipid present in all cell membranes. It has an important role in fat transport and is the precursor from which bile salts and adrenal and sex hormones are made.

Dietary fats consist mainly of triglycerides, which can be split into glycerol and chains of carbon, hydrogen and oxygen called fatty acids. This action, the digestion or breakdown of fats, is achieved in the human intestine by enzymes known as lipases, which are present primarily in the pancreatic and intestinal secretions. Bile salts from the liver emulsify the fatty acids to make them more soluble in water and hence more easily absorbed.

The many fatty acids in human diets are divided into two main groups: saturated and unsaturated. The latter group includes both polyunsaturated and mono-unsaturated fatty acids. Saturated fatty acids have the maximum number of hydrogen atoms that their chemical structure will permit. All fats and oils eaten by humans are mixtures of saturated and unsaturated fatty acids. Broadly speaking, fats from land animals (i.e. meat fat, butter and ghee) contain more saturated fatty acids than do those of vegetable origin. Fats from plant products and to some extent those from fish have more unsaturated fatty acids, particularly polyunsaturated fatty acids (PUFAs).There are exceptions, however. For example, coconut oil has a large amount of saturated fatty acids.

These groupings of fats have important health implications because excess intake of saturated fats is one of the risk factors associated with arteriosclerosis and coronary heart disease. In contrast, PUFAs are believed to be protective.

PUFAs also include two unsaturated fatty acids, linoleic acid and linolenic acid, which have been termed 'essential fatty acids' (EFAs) as they are necessary for good health. EFAs are important in the synthesis of many cell structures and several biologically important compounds. Recent studies have also shown the benefits of other longer-chain fatty acids in the growth and development of young children, and arachidonic acid and docosa-hexaenoicacid (OHA) should conditionally be considered essential during early development. Experiments with animals and studies in humans have shown definite skin and growth changes and abnormal vascular and neural function in the absence of these fatty acids, and there is no doubt that they are essential for the nutrition of individual cells and tissues of the body.

Fat is desirable to make the diet more palatable. It also yields about 9 kcal/g, which is more than twice the energy yielded by carbohydrates and proteins (about 4 kcal/g); fat can therefore reduce the bulk of the diet. A person doing very heavy work, especially in a cold climate, may require as many as 4 000 kcal a day. In such a case it is highly desirable that a good proportion of the energy should come from fat; otherwise the diet would be very bulky. Bulky diets can be a particularly serious problem in young children as well. A reasonable increase in the fat or oil content of the diets of young children raises the energy density of predominantly bulky carbohydrate diets and is highly desirable.

Fat also functions as a vehicle that assists the absorption of fat-soluble vitamins.

Thus fats, and even specific types of fat, are essential to health. However, practically all diets provide the small amount required.

Fat deposited in the human body serves as a reserve fuel. It is an economic way of storing energy, because, fat yields about twice as much energy, weight for weight, as does carbohydrate or protein. Fat is present beneath the skin as an insulation against cold, and it forms a supporting tissue for many organs such as the heart and intestines.

All fat in the body is not necessarily derived from fat that has been eaten. However, excess calories from the carbohydrate and protein in, for example, maize, cassava, rice or wheat can be converted into fat in the human body.

Proteins

Like carbohydrates and fats, proteins contain carbon, hydrogen and oxygen, but they also contain nitrogen and often sulphur. They are particularly important as nitrogenous substances, and are necessary for growth and repair of the body. Proteins are the main structural constituents of the cells and tissues of the body, and they make up the greater portion of the substance of the muscles and organs (apart from water). The proteins in different body tissues are not all exactly the same. The proteins in liver, in blood and in specific hormones, for example, are all different.

Proteins are necessary–

- For growth and development of the body;
- For body maintenance and the repair and replacement of worn out or damaged tissues;
- To produce metabolic and digestive enzymes;
- As an essential constituent of certain hormones, such as thyroxine and insulin.

Although proteins can yield energy, their main importance is rather as an essential constituent of all cells. All cells may need replacement from time to time, and their replacement requires protein.

Any protein eaten in excess of the amount needed for growth, cell and fluid replacement and various other metabolic functions is used to provide energy, which the body obtains by changing the protein into carbohydrate. If the carbohydrate and fat in the diet do not provide adequate energy, then protein is used to provide energy; as a result less protein is available for growth, cell replacement and other metabolic needs. This point is especially important for children, who need extra protein for growth. If they get too little food for their energy requirements, then the protein will be diverted for daily energy needs and will not be used for growth.

Amino Acids

All proteins consist of large molecules which are made of amino acids. The amino acids in any protein are linked together in chains, called peptide linkages. The various proteins are made of different amino acids linked together in different chains. Becausethere are many different amino acids, there are many different possible configurations, so there are many different proteins.

During digestion proteins break down to form amino acids much as complex carbohydrates such as starches break down into simple monosaccharides and fats break down into fatty acids. In the stomach and intestines various proteolytic enzymes hydrolyse the protein, releasing amino acids and peptides.

Plants are able to synthesize amino acids from simple inorganic chemical substances. Animals do not have this ability; they derive all the amino acids necessary for building their protein from consumption of plants or animals. As the animals eaten by humans initially derived their protein from plants, all amino acids in human diets have originated from this source.

Animals have differing abilities to convert one amino acid into another. In the human this ability is limited. Conversion occurs mainly in the liver. If the ability to convert one amino acid into another were unlimited, then the question of the protein content of diets and the prevention of protein deficiency would be simple. It would be enough merely to supply sufficient protein, irrespective of the quality or amino acid content of the protein supplied.

Of the large number of amino acids, 20 are common in plants and animals. Of these, eight have been found to be essential for the adult human and have thus been termed 'essential amino acids' or 'indispensable amino acids', namely: phenyl-alanine, tryptophan, methionine, lysine, leucine, isoleucine,valine and threonine. A ninth amino acid, histidine, is required for growth and is essential for infants and children; it may also be necessary for tissue repair. Other amino acids include glycine, alanine, serine, cystine, tyrosine, aspartic acid, glutamic acid, proline, hydroxyproline, citrulline and arginine. Each protein in a food is composed of a particular mixture of amino acids which might or might not contain all eight of the essential ones.

Protein Quality and Quantity

To assess the protein value of any food it is useful to know how much total protein it contains, which amino acids it has and how many essential amino acids are present and in what proportion. Much is now known about the individual proteins present in various foods, their amino acid content and therefore their quality and quantity. Some have a better mixture of amino acids than others, and these are said to have a higher biological value. The proteins albumin in egg and casein in milk, for example, contain all the essential amino acids in good proportions and are nutritionally superior to such proteins as zein in maize, which contains little tryptophan or lysine, and the protein in wheat, which contains only small quantities of lysine. It is not true, however, to say that the proteins in maize and wheat are not valuable. Although they contain less of certain amino acids, they do contain some amount of all the essential amino acids as well as many of the other important ones. The relative deficiency of maize and wheat proteins can be overcome by providing other foodstuffs containing more of the limited amino acids. It is therefore possible for two foods with low-value protein to complement each other to form a good protein mixture when eaten together.

Humans, especially children on diets deficient in animal protein, require a variety of foods of vegetable origin, not just one staple food. In many diets, pulses or legumes such as groundnuts, beans and cowpeas, though short of sulphur-containing amino acids, supplement the cereal proteins, which are often short of lysine. A mixture of foods of vegetable origin, especially if taken at the same meal, can serve as a substitute for animal protein.

FAO has produced tables showing the content of essential amino acids in different foodstuffs, from which it can be seen which foods best complement each other. It is also necessary, of course, to ascertain the total quantity of protein and amino acids in any food.

The quality of the protein depends largely on its amino acid composition and its digestibility. If a protein is deficient in one or more essential amino acids, its quality is lower. The most deficient of the essential amino acids in a protein is called the 'limiting amino acid'. The limiting amino acid determines the efficiency of utilization of the protein present in a food or combination of foods. Human beings usually eat food in meals which contain many proteins; they seldom consume just one protein. Therefore nutritionists are interested in the protein quality of a person's diet or meals, rather than just one food. If one essential amino acid is in short supply in the diet, it limits the use of the other amino acids for building protein.

Readers who wish to become familiar with the methods used for determining protein quality are advised to consult comprehensive textbooks on nutrition, which describe them in detail. One method uses experiments on growth and nitrogen retention in young rats. Another involves determination of the amino acid or chemical score, usually by examining the efficiency of utilization of proteins in the foods consumed by comparing their amino acid composition with that of protein known to be of high quality, such as that in whole eggs.

The chemical score may thus be defined as the efficiency of utilization of food protein in comparison with whole egg protein. Net Protein Utilization (NPU) is a measure of the amount or percentage of protein retained in relation to that consumed. As an example, Table below gives the chemical score and NPU of the protein in five foods.

It is not usual or easy to obtain NPU values in people, and in most studies rats are used. Table 16 suggests that there is a good correlation between the values in rats and in children, and that chemical score provides a reasonable estimate of protein quality.

For the professional involved in nutritional activities to help people–be it a dietitian in a health facility, an agricultural extension worker or a nutrition educator what is important is that the protein value differs among foods and that mixing foods improves the protein quality of the meal or the diet. Table 17 gives the protein content and the limiting amino acid score of some commonly eaten plant-based foods. Because lysine is most commonly the limiting amino acid in many foods of plant origin, the lysine score is also given.

Protein Digestion and Absorption

Proteins consumed in the diet undergo a series of chemical changes in the gastrointestinal tract. The physiology of protein digestion is complicated; pepsin and rennin from the stomach, trypsin from the pancreas and erepsin from the intestines hydrolyse proteins into their component amino acids. Most of the amino acids are absorbed into the bloodstream from the small intestine and thus travel to the liver and from there all over the body. Any surplus amino acids are stripped of the amino (NH2) group, which goes to form urea in the urine, leaving the rest of the molecule to be transformed into glucose. There is now some evidence that a little intact protein is taken up into certain cells lining thc intestines. Some of this protein in the infant may have a role in the passive immunity conveyed from the mother to her newborn child.

A little of the protein and amino acids released in the intestines is not absorbed. The unabsorbed amino acids, plus cells shed from the intestinal villi and acted upon by bacteria, together with gut organisms, contribute to the nitrogen found in faeces.

Table: Chemical Score and Net Protein Utilization in Selected Foods

Food	Chemical Score	NPU Determined in Children	NPU Determined in Rats
Eggs (whole)	100	87	94
Milk (human)	100	94	87
Rice	67	63	59

Food	Chemical Score	NPU Determined in Children	NPU Determined in Rats
Maize	49	36	52
Wheat	53	49	48

Table: Protein Content, Limiting Amino Acid Score and Lysine Score of Selected Plant Foods

Food	Protein Content (%)	Limiting Amino Add Score	Lysine score
		Cereals	
Maize	9.4	49 (Lys)	49
Rice (white)	7.1	62 (Lys)	62
Wheat flour	10.3	38 (Lys)	38
Millet	11.0	33 (Lys)	33
		Legumes	
Kidney beans	23.6	100	118
Cowpea	23.5	100	117
Groundnut	25.8	62 (Lys)	62
		Vegetables	
Tomato	0.9	56 (Leu)	64
Squash	1.2	70 (Thr)	95
Pepper, sweet	0.9	77 (Lys Leu)	77
Cassava	1.3	44 (Leu)	56
Potato	2.1	91 (Leu)	105

Much of the protein in the human body is present in muscle. There is no true storage of protein in the body as there is with fat and to a small extent glycogen. However, there is now little doubt that a well-nourished individual has sufficient protein accumulated to be able to last several days without replenishment and to remain still in good health.

Protein Requirements

Children need more protein than adults because they need to grow. Infants in the first few months of life require about 2.5 g of protein per kilogram of body weight. This requirement drops to about 1.5 g/kg at nine to 12 months of age. Unless energy intakes are adequate, however, the protein will not all be used for growth. A pregnant woman needs an additional supply of protein to build up the foetus inside her. Similarly, a lactating woman needs extra protein, because the milk she secretes contains protein. In some societies it is common for women to breastfeed their babies for as long as two years. Thus some women need extra protein for two years and nine months for every infant they bear.

Protein requirements and recommended allowances have been the subject of much research, debate and disagreement over the past 50 years.

The safe level of intake for a one-year-old child was put at 1.5 g per kilogram of body weight. The amount then falls to 1 g/kg at age six years. The US recommended dietary allowance (RDA) is a little higher, namely 1.75g/kg at age one year and 1.2g/kg at age six years. In adults the safe intake of protein is 0.8 g/kg for females and 0.85 g/kg for males.

The safe levels of intake of protein by age and gender, including those for pregnant and lactating women, are given in Chapter 8. Values are provided both for a diet high in fibre, comprising mainly cereals, roots and legumes with little food of animal origin, and for a mixed balanced diet with less fibre and plenty of complete protein. As an example, a non pregnant adult woman weighing 55 kg requires 49 g of protein per day for the first diet and 41 g per day for the second. Fibre reduces protein utilization.

Inadequate protein intake jeopardizes growth and repair in the body. Protein deficiency is especially dangerous for children because they are growing and also because the risk of infection is greater during childhood than at almost any other time of life. In children inadequate energy intake also has an impact on protein, in the absence of adequate energy some protein needs to be diverted and therefore will not be used for growth.

In many developing countries (though not all), the intake of protein is relatively low and of predominantly vegetable origin. The paucity of foods of animal origin in the diet is not always a matter of choice. For example, many low-income Africans and Latin Americans like animal products but find them less freely available, more difficult to produce and store and more expensive than most vegetable products. Diets low in meat, fish and dairy products are very common in countries where most people are poor.

Infections lead to an increased loss of nitrogen from the body, which has to be replaced by proteins in the diet. Therefore children and others who have frequent infections will have greater protein needs than healthy persons. This fact must constantly be borne in mind, for in developing countries many children suffer an almost continual series of infectious diseases; they may frequently get diarrhoea, and they may harbour intestinal parasites.

Minerals

Minerals have a number of functions in the body. Sodium, potassium and chlorine are present as salts in body fluids, where they have a physiological role in maintaining osmotic pressure. Minerals form part of the constitution of many tissues. For example, calcium and phosphorus in bones combine to give rigidity to the whole body. Minerals are present in body acids and alkalis; for example, chlorine occurs in hydrochloric acid in the stomach. They are also essential constituents of certain hormones, e.g. iodine in the thyroxine produced by the thyroid gland.

The principal minerals in the human body are calcium, phosphorus, potassium, sodium, chlorine, sulphur, copper, magnesium, manganese, iron, iodine, fluorine, zinc, cobalt and selenium. Phosphorus is so widely available in plants that a shortage of this element is unlikely in any diet. Potassium, sodium and chlorine are easily absorbed and are physiologically more important than phosphorus. Sulphur is consumed by humans mainly in the form of sulphur-containing amino acids; thus sulphur deficiency, when it occurs, is linked with protein deficiency. Copper, manganese and magnesium deficiencies are not believed to be common. The minerals that are of most importance in human nutrition are thus calcium, iron, iodine, fluorine and zinc, and only these are discussed in some detail here. Some mineral elements are required in very tiny amounts in human diets but are still vital for metabolic purposes; these are termed essential trace elements.

The table giving the nutrient content of selected foods shows the relative content of some important minerals in different foods.

Calcium

The body of an average-sized adult contains about 1,250 g of calcium. Over 99 per cent of the calcium is in the bones and teeth, where it is combined with phosphorus as calcium phosphate, a hard substance that gives the body rigidity. However, although hard and rigid, the skeleton of the body is not the unchanging structure it appears to be. In fact, the bones are a cellular matrix, and the calcium is continuously taken up by the bones and given back to the body. The bones, therefore, serve as a reserve supply of this mineral.

Calcium is present in the serum of the blood in small but important quantities, usually about 10 mg per 100 ml of serum. There are also about 10 g of calcium in the extracellular fluids and soft tissues of the adult body.

Properties and Functions

In humans and other mammals, calcium and phosphorus together have an important role as major components of the skeleton. They are also important, however, in metabolic functions such as muscular function, nervous stimuli, enzymatic and hormonal activities and transport of oxygen. These functions are described in detail in textbooks of physiology and nutrition.

The skeleton of a living person is physiologically different from the dry skeleton in a grave or museum. The bones are living tissues, consisting mainly of a mineralized protein collagen substance. In the living body there is continuous turnover of calcium. Bone is laid down and resorbed all the time, in people of all ages. Bone cells called osteoclasts take up or resorb bone, while others, termed osteoblasts, lay down or form new bone. The bone cells in the mineralized collagen are called osteocytes.

Up to full growth or maturity (which has usually taken place by age 18 to 22 years), new bone is formed as the skeleton enlarges to its adult size. In young adults, despite bone re-modelling, the skeleton generally maintains its size. However, as persons get older there is some loss of bone mass.

A complex physiological system maintains proper calcium and phosphorus levels. The control involves hormones from the parathyroid gland, calcitonin and the active form of vitamin D (l,25-dihydroxy cholecalciferol).

Small but highly important amounts of calcium are present in extracellular fluids, particularly blood plasma, as well as in various body cells. In serum most of the calcium is in two forms, ionized and protein bound. Laboratories usually measure only total plasma calcium; the normal range is 8.5 to 10.5 mg/dl (2.1 to 2.6 mmol/litre). A drop in the level of calcium to below 2.1 mmol/litre is termed hypocalcaemia and can lead to various symptoms. Tetany (not to be confused with tetanus resulting from the tetanus bacillus), characterized by spasms and sometimes fits, results from low levels of ionized calcium in the blood.

Dietary Sources

All the calcium in the body, except that inherited from the mother, comes from food and water consumed. It is especially necessary to have adequate quantities of calcium during growth, for it is at this stage that the bones develop.

The foetus in the mother's uterus has most of its nutritional requirements satisfied, for in terms of nutrition the unborn child is almost parasitic. If the mother's diet is poor in calcium, she draws extra supplies of this mineral from her bones.

An entirely breastfed infant will obtain adequate calcium from breastmilk as long as the volume of milk is sufficient. Contrary to popular belief, the calcium content of human milk varies rather little; 100 ml of breastmilk, even from an undernourished mother on a diet very low in calcium, provides approximately 30 mg of calcium. A lactating mother secreting 1 litre will thus lose 300 mg of calcium per day.

Cow's milk is a very rich source of calcium, richer than human milk. Whereas a litre of human milk contains 300 mg of calcium, a litre of cow's milk contains 1200 mg. The difference arises because a cow has to provide for her calf, which grows much more rapidly than a human infant and needs extra calcium for the hardening of its fast-growing skeleton. Similarly, the milk of most other domestic animals has a higher calcium content than human milk. This does not mean, however, that a child would be better off drinking cow's milk rather than human milk. Cow's milk yields more calcium than a child needs. A child (or even a baby) who drinks large quantities of cow's milk excretes any excess calcium, so it is of no benefit; it does not increase the child's growth rate beyond what is optimal.

Milk products such as cheese and yoghurt are also rich sources of calcium. Small saltwater and freshwater fish such as sardines and sprats supply good quantities of calcium since they are usually eaten whole, bones and all. Small dried fish add useful calcium to the diet. Vegetables and pulses provide some calcium. Although cereals and roots are relatively poor sources of calcium, they often supply the major portion of the mineral in tropical diets by virtue of the quantities consumed.

Table: Calcium Content of Various Milks

Source of Milk	**Calcium Content *(mg/100 ml)***
Human	32
Cow	119
Camel	120
Goat	134
Water buffalo	169
Sheep	193

The calcium content of drinking-water varies from place to place. Hard water usually contains high levels of calcium.

Absorption and Utilization

The absorption of calcium is variable and generally rather low. It is related to the absorption of phosphorus and the other important mineral constituents of the bones. Vitamin D is essential for the proper absorption of calcium. Thus a person seriously deficient in vitamin D absorbs too little calcium, even if the intake of calcium is more than adequate, and could have a negative calcium balance. Phytates, phosphates and oxalates in food reduce calcium absorption.

Persons customarily consuming diets low in calcium appear to have better absorption of calcium than those on high-calcium diets. Unabsorbed calcium is excreted in the faeces. Excess calcium is excreted in the urine and in sweat.

Requirements

It is not easy to state categorically the human requirements for calcium, because there are several factors influencing absorption and considerable variations in calcium losses among individuals.

Needs for calcium are increased during pregnancy and lactation, and children require more calcium because of growth. Those on high-protein diets require more calcium in the diet.

The following are recommended levels of daily calcium intake:

- Adults, 400 to 500 mg;
- Children, 400 to 700 mg;
- Pregnant and lactating women, 800 to 1 000 mg.

Deficiency States

Disease or malformation caused primarily by dietary deficiency of calcium is rare. There is little convincing evidence to show that the many diets of adults in developing countries supplying perhaps only 250 to 300 mg of calcium daily are harmful to health. It is assumed that adults achieve some sort of balance when intakes of calcium are low. Females who go through a series of pregnancies and long lactations may lose calcium and be at risk of osteomalacia. However, vitamin D deficiency, not calcium deficiency, is more often implicated in this condition. In children the development of rickets results from vitamin D deficiency, not from dietary lack of calcium, in spite of increased calcium requirements in childhood. Calcium balance in childhood is generally positive, and calcium deficiency has not been shown to have an adverse influence on growth.

Osteoporosis is a common disease of ageing, especially in women. The skeleton becomes demineralized, which leads to fragility of bones and commonly to fractures of the hip, vertebrae and other bones, particularly in older women. High calcium intake is often recommended but has not been proved effective in prevention and/or treatment.

Exercise appears to reduce the loss of calcium from bones; this may explain, in part, why osteoporosis is less prevalent in many developing countries, where women work hard and are very active. There is now clear evidence that providing the female hormone Oestrogen to women after menopause reduces bone loss and osteoporosis.

Iron

Iron deficiency is a very common cause of ill health in all parts of the world, both South and North. The average iron content in a healthy adult is only about 3 to 4 g, yet this relatively small quantity is vital.

Properties and Functions

Most of the iron in the body is present in the red blood cells, mainly as a component of haemoglobin. Much of the rest is present in myoglobin, a compound occurring mainly in muscles, and as storage iron or ferritin, mainly in the liver, spleen and bone marrow. Additional tiny quantities are found binding protein in the blood plasma and in respiratory enzymes.

The main, vital function of iron is in the transfer of oxygen at various sites in the body. Haemoglobin is the pigment in the erythrocytes that carries oxygen from the lungs to the tissues. Myoglobin in skeletal and heart muscle accepts the oxygen from the haemoglobin. Iron is also present in peroxidase, catalase and the cytochromes.

Iron is an element that is neither used up nor destroyed in the properly functioning body. Unlike some minerals, it is not required for excretion, and only very small amounts appear in urine and sweat. Minute quantities are lost in desquamated cells from the skin and intestine, in shed hair and nails and in the bile and other body secretions.

The body is, however, efficient, economical and conservative in the use of iron. Iron released when the erythrocytes are old and broken down is taken up and used again and again for the manufacture of new erythrocytes. This economy of iron is important. In normal circumstances, only about 1 mg of iron is lost from the body daily by excretion into the intestines, in urine, in sweat or through loss of hair or surface epithelial cells.

Because iron is conserved, the nutritional needs of healthy males and postmenopausal females are very small. Women of child-bearing age, however, must replace the iron lost during menstruation and childbirth and must meet the additional requirements of pregnancy and lactation. Children have relatively high needs because of their rapid growth, which involves increases not only in body size but also in blood volume.

Dietary Sources

Iron is present in a variety of foods of both plant and animal origin. Rich food sources include meat (especially liver), fish, eggs, legumes (including a variety of beans, peas and other pulses) and green leafy vegetables. Cereal grains such as maize, rice and wheat contain moderate amounts of iron, but because these are often staple foods and eaten in large quantities, they provide most of the iron for many people, in developing countries. Iron cooking pots may be a source of iron.

Milk, contrary to the notion that it is the 'complete food,' is a poor source of iron. Human milk contains about 2 mg of iron per litre and cow's milk only half this amount.

Absorption and Utilization

Absorption of iron takes place mainly in the upper portion of the small intestine. Most of the iron enters the bloodstream directly and not through the lymphatic system. Evidence indicates that absorption is regulated to some extent by physiological demand. Persons who are iron deficient tend to absorb iron more efficiently and in greater quantities than do normal subjects.

Several other factors affect iron absorption. For example, tannins, phosphates and phytates in food reduce iron absorption, whereas ascorbic acid increases it. Studies have indicated that egg yolk, despite its relatively high iron content, inhibits absorption of iron - not only the iron from the egg yolk itself, but also that from other foods.

Healthy subjects normally absorb only 5 to 10 per cent of the iron in their foods, whereas iron-deficient subjects may absorb twice that amount. Therefore, on a diet that supplies 15 mg of iron, the normal person would absorb 0.75 to 1.5 mg of iron, but the iron-deficient person would absorb as much as

3 mg. Iron absorption generally increases during growth and pregnancy, after bleeding and in other conditions in which the demand for iron is enhanced.

Of greatest importance is the fact that the availability of iron from foods varies widely. Absorption of the haem iron in foods of animal origin (meat, fish and poultry) is usually very high, whereas the non-haem iron in foods such as cereals, vegetables, roots and fruits is poorly absorbed.

However, people usually eat meals, not single individual foods, and a small amount of haem iron consumed with a meal where most of the iron is non-haem iron will enhance the absorption of all the iron. Thus the addition of a quite small amount of haem iron from perhaps fish or meat to a large helping of rice or maize containing non-haem iron will result in much greater absorption of iron from the cereal staple. If this meal also includes fruits or vegetables, the vitamin C in them will also enhance iron absorption. However, if tea is consumed with this meal, the tannin present in the tea will reduce the absorption of iron.

The dietary requirements for iron are approximately ten times the body's physiological requirements. If a normally healthy man or post menopausal woman requires 1 mg of iron daily because of iron losses, then the dietary requirements are about 10 mg per day. This recommendation allows a fair margin of safety, as absorption is increased with need. Menstrual loss of iron has been estimated to average a little less than 1 mg per day during an entire year. It is recommended that women of child-bearing age have a dietary intake of 18 mg per day.

During pregnancy, the body requires on average about 1.5 mg of iron daily to develop the foetus and supportive tissues and to expand the maternal blood supply. Most of this additional iron is required in the second and third trimesters of pregnancy.

Breastfeeding women use iron to provide the approximately 2 mg of iron per litre of breastmilk. However, during the first six to 15 months of intensive breastfeeding they may not menstruate, so they do not lose iron in menstrual blood.

Newborn infants are born with very high haemoglobin levels (a high red blood cell count), termed polycythaemia, which provides an extra store of iron. This iron, together with that present in breastmilk, is usually sufficient for the first four to six months of life, after which iron from other foods becomes necessary.

Premature and other low-birth-weight infants may have lower iron stores and be at greater risk than other infants.

An excess intake of iron over long periods can lead to the disease siderosis or haemachromatosis. This disease is reported to occur most commonly where beer or other alcoholic beverages are brewed in iron cooking pots, particularly in South Africa. In alcoholics siderosis leading to iron deposits in the liver may be associated with cirrhosis.

Deficiency States

Consideration of the iron requirements and the iron content of commonly eaten foods might suggest that iron deficiency is rare, but this is not the case. Food iron is poorly absorbed. Iron is not readily excreted into the urine or the gastro-intestinal tract; thus severe iron deficiency is usually associated with an increased need for iron resulting from conditions such as pregnancy, blood loss or expansion of the total body mass during growth. Iron deficiency is most common in young children, in women of child-bearing age and in persons with chronic blood loss. The end result of iron deficiency is anaemia.

Hookworm infections, which are extremely prevalent in many countries, result in loss of blood which may cause iron deficiency anaemia. In some parts of the tropics schistosomiasis is also common, and this disease also causes blood loss.

Iodine

The body of an average adult contains about 20 to 50 mg of iodine, much of it in the thyroid gland. Iodine is essential for the formation of thyroid hormones secreted by this gland.

Properties and Functions

In humans iodine functions as an essential component of the hormones of the thyroid gland, an endocrine gland situated in the lower neck. Thyroid hormones, of which the most important is thyroxine (T4), are important for regulating metabolism.

In children they support normal growth and development, including mental development.

Iodine is absorbed from the gut as iodide, and excess is excreted in the urine. The adult thyroid gland, in a person consuming adequate iodine, traps about 60 flg of iodine per day to make normal amounts of thyroid hormones. If there is insufficient iodine, the thyroid works harder to trap more; the gland enlarges in size (a condition known as goitre), and its iodine content might become markedly reduced.

Thyroid stimulating hormone (TSH) from the pituitary gland influences thyroxine secretion and iodine trapping. In severe iodine deficiency, TSH levels are raised and thyroxine levels are low.

Dietary Sources

Iodine is widely present in rocks and soils. The quantity in different plants varies according to the soil in which they are grown. It is not meaningful to list the iodine content of foodstuffs because of the large variations in iodine content from place to place, depending on the iodine content of the soil. Iodine tends to get washed out of the soil, and throughout the ages a considerable quantity has flowed into the sea. Sea fish, seaweed and most vegetables grown near the sea are useful sources of iodine. Drinking-water provides some iodine but very seldom enough to satisfy human requirements.

In many countries where goitre is prevalent the authorities have added iodine to salt, a strategy which has successfully controlled iodine deficiency disorders (IDD). Iodine has usually been added to salt in the form of potassium iodide, but another form, potassium iodate, is more stable and is better in hot, humid climates. Iodated salt is an important dietary source of iodine.

Deficiency States

A lack of iodine in the diet results in several health problems, one of which is goitre, or enlargement of the thyroid gland. Goitre is extremely prevalent in many countries. There are other contributing causes of goitre, but iodine deficiency is by far the most common-Iodinedeficiency during pregnancy may lead to cretinism, mental retardation and other problems, which may be permanent, in the child. It is now known that endemic goitre and cretinism are not the only problems caused by iodine deficiency. The decrease in mental capacity associated with iodine deficiency is of particular concern.

Fluorine

Fluorine is a mineral element found mainly in the teeth and skeleton. Traces of fluorine in the teeth help to protect them against decay. Fluorides consumed during childhood become a part of the dental enamel and make it more resistant to the weak organic acids formed from foods that adhere to or get stuck between the teeth. This strengthening greatly reduces the chances of decay or caries developing in the teeth. Some studies have suggested that fluoride may also help strengthen bone, particularly later in life, and may thus inhibit the development of osteoporosis.

Dietary Sources

The main source of fluorine for most human beings is the water they drink. If the water has a fluorine content of about one part per million (1 ppm), then it will supply adequate fluorine for the teeth. However, many water supplies contain much less than this amount. Fluorine is present in bone; consequently small fish that are consumed whole are a good source. Tea has a high fluorine content. Few other foods contain much fluorine.

Deficiency

If the fluoride content of drinking-water in any locality is below 0.5 ppm, dental caries will probably be much more prevalent than where the concentration is higher.

The recommended level of fluoride in water is between 0.8 and 1.2 ppm. In some countries or localities where the content of fluorine in the water is less than 1 ppm, it has now become the practice to add fluoride to the water supply.

This practice is strongly recommended, but it is only practicable for large piped-water supplies; in some developing countries where most people do not have piped water, it is not feasible. The addition of fluoride to toothpaste also helps reduce dental caries. Fluorine does not totally prevent dental caries, but it can reduce the incidence by 60 to 70 per cent.

Excess

An excessively high intake of fluoride causes a condition known as dental fluorosis, in which the teeth become mottled.

It is usually caused by consuming excessive fluoride in water supplies that have high fluoride levels. In some parts of Africa and Asia, natural waters contain over 4 ppm of fluoride. Very high fluorine intakes also cause bone changes with sclerosis (added bone density), calcification of muscle insertions and exostoses. Skeletal fluorosis can cause severe pain and serious bone abnormalities.

Zinc

Zinc is an essential element in human nutrition, and its importance to human health has received much recent attention. Zinc is present in many important enzymes essential for metabolism. The body of a healthy human adult contains 2 to 3 g of zinc and requires around 15 mg of dietary zinc per day. Most of the zinc in the body is in the skeleton, but other tissues (such as the skin and hair) and some organs (particularly the prostate) have relatively high concentrations.

Dietary Sources

Zinc is present in most foods both of vegetable and of animal origin, but the richest sources tend to be protein-rich foods such as meat, seafoods and eggs. In developing countries, however, where most people consume relatively small amounts of these foods, most zinc comes from cereal grains and legumes.

Absorption and Utilization

As with iron, absorption of zinc from the diet is inhibited by food constituents such as phytates, oxalate and tannins. No simple tests of human zinc status are known, however. Indicators used include evidence of low dietary intake, low blood serum zinc levels and low quantities of zinc in hair specimens.

Much research on this mineral has been undertaken in the last two decades, and a great deal of knowledge concerning zinc metabolism and zinc deficiency in animals and humans has been gathered. Nonetheless, there is little evidence to suggest that zinc deficiency is an important public health problem for large numbers of people in any country, industrialized or developing. However, research now under way may show that poor zinc status is responsible for poor growth, reduced appetite and other conditions; in this way zinc deficiency may contribute especially to what is now called protein-energy malnutrition (PEM).

Zinc deficiency is responsible for a very rare congenital disease known as acrodermatitis enteropathica. It responds to zinc therapy. Some patients receiving all of their nutrients intravenously have developed skin lesions which also respond to zinc treatment. In the Near East, particularly in the Islamic Republic of Iran and Egypt, a condition has been described in which adolescent or near-adolescent boys are dwarfed and have poorly developed genitalia and delayed onset of puberty; this condition has been said to respond to zinc treatment.

Zinc deficiency has also been reported as secondary to, or as a part of, other conditions such as PEM, various malabsorption conditions, alcoholism including cirrhosis of the liver, renal disease and metabolic disorders.

Other Trace Elements

Numerous minerals are present in the human body. For most of the trace elements, there is no evidence that deficiency is responsible for major public health problems anywhere. Some of these minerals are very important in metabolism or as constituents of body tissues. Many of them have been studied, and their chemistry and biochemistry have been described. Experimental deficiencies have been produced in laboratory animals, but most human diets, even poor diets, do not appear to lead to important deficiencies. These minerals therefore are not of public health importance. Other trace elements are present in the body but do not have any known essential role. Some minerals, for example lead and mercury, are of great interest to health workers because excess intake has commonly resulted in toxic manifestations.

Cobalt, copper, magnesium, manganese and selenium deserve mention because of their important nutritional role, and lead and mercury because of their toxicity. These minerals are considered in detail in large comprehensive textbooks of nutrition.

Cobalt

Cobalt is of interest to nutritionists because it is an essential part of vitamin B12 (cyanocobalamin). When isolated as a crystalline substance, the vitamin was found to contain about 4 per cent cobalt. However, cobalt deficiency does not play a part in the anaemia that results from vitamin B12 deficiency.

Copper

Copper deficiency is known to cause anaemia in cattle, but no such risk is known in adult humans.

Some evidence suggests that copper deficiency leads to anaemia in premature infants, in people with severe PEM and in those maintained on parenteral nutrition. An extremely rare congenital condition known as Menkes' disease is caused by failure of copper absorption.

Magnesium

Magnesium is an essential mineral present mainly in the bones but also in most human tissues. Most diets contain adequate dietary magnesium, but under some circumstances, such as diarrhoea, severe PEM and other conditions, excessive body losses of magnesium occur. Such losses may lead to weakness and mental changes and occasionally to convulsions.

Selenium

Both deficiency and excess of Selenium have been well described in livestock. In areas of China where the soil is low in selenium, therefore the food composition of selenium, is low. A heart condition has been described; termed Keshan's disease, it is a serious condition affecting heart muscle. Chinese researchers believe it can be prevented by providing dietary selenium. Selenium deficiency has also been associated with certain cancers.

Lead

Lead is of great public health importance because it commonly causes toxicity. Human lead deficiency is not known. Lead poisoning is especially an urban problem and is most important in children. It may lead to neurological and mental problems and to anaemia. Excess lead intake may result from consumption of lead in the household (from lead-based paint or water pipes containing lead) and from intake of atmospheric lead (from motor vehicle emissions).

Mercury

Mercury deficiency is not known in humans. The concern is with excessively high intakes of mercury and the risks of toxicity, Fish in waters contaminated with mercury concentrate the mineral There is a danger of toxicity in those who consume fish with high mercury content.

Mercury poisoning resulting from consumption of seeds coated with a mercury-containing fungicide has been described in Asia, Latin America and the Near East. The effects include severe neurological symptoms and paralysis.

Vitamins

Vitamins are organic substances present in minute amounts in foodstuffs and necessary for metabolism. They are grouped together not because they are chemically related or have similar physiological functions, but because, as their name implies, they are vital factors in the diet and because they were all discovered in connection with the diseases resulting from their deficiency.

Moreover, they do not fit into the other nutrient categories (carbohydrates, fats, protein and minerals or trace metals).

When vitamins were first being classified, each was named after a letter of the alphabet. Subsequently, there has been a tendency to drop the letters in favour of chemical names. The use of the chemical name is justified when the vitamin has a known chemical formula, as with the main vitamins of the B group. Nevertheless, it is advantageous to include certain vitamins under group headings, even if they are not chemically related, since they do tend to occur in the same foodstuffs.

·In this only vitamin A, five of the B vitamins (thiamine, riboflavin, niacin, vitamin B12 and folic acid), vitamin C and vitamin D are described in detail. Other vitamins known to be vital to health include pantothenic acid (of which a deficiency may cause the burning feet syndrome mentioned below), biotin (vitamin H), para-aminobenzoic acid, choline, vitamin E and vitamin K (antihaemorrhagic vitamin).

Vitamin A (Retinol)

Vitamin A was discovered in 1913 when research workers found that certain laboratory animals stopped growing when lard (made from pork fat) was the only form of tat present in their diet, whereas when butter was supplied instead of lard (with the diet remaining otherwise the same) the animals grew and thrived. Further animal experiments showed that egg yolk and cod-liver oil contained the same vital food factor, which was named vitamin A.

It was later established that many vegetable products had the same nutritional properties as the vitamin A in butter; they were found to contain a yellow pigment called carotene, some of which can be converted to vitamin A in the human body.

Properties

Retinol is the main form of vitamin A in human diets. (Retinol is the chemical name of the alcohol derivative, and it is used as the reference standard.) In its pure crystalline form, retinol is a very pale yellow-green substance. It is soluble in fat but insoluble in water, and it is found only in animal products. Other forms of vitamin A exist, but they have somewhat different molecular configurations and less biological activity than retinol, and they are not important in human diets.

Carotenes, which act as provitamins or precursors of vitamin A, are yellow substances that occur widely in plant substances. In some foodstuffs their colour may be masked by the green plant pigment chlorophyll, which often occurs in close association with carotenes. There are several different carotenes. One of these, beta-carotene, is the most important source of vitamin A in the diets of most people living in non industrialized countries. The other carotenes, or carotenoids, have little or no nutritional importance for humans. In the past, food analyses have often failed to distinguish beta-carotene from other carotenes.

Vitamin A is an important component of the visual purple of the retina of the eye, and if vitamin A is deficient, the ability to see in dim light is reduced. This condition is called night blindness. The biochemical basis for the other lesions of vitamin A deficiency has not been fully explained. The main change, in pathological terms, is a keratinizing metaplasia which is seen on various epithelial surfaces. Vitamin A appears to be necessary for the protection of surface tissue.

Several studies have shown that adequate vitamin A status reduces infant and child mortality in certain populations. Vitamin A supplementation reduces case fatality rates from measles. In other illnesses such as diarrhoea and respiratory infections, however, there is not strong evidence that the prevalence or duration of morbidity is reduced by vitamin A dosing.

Calculating Vitamin A Content In Foods

1 IV retinol = 0.3 flg retinol = 0.3 RE
1 RE = 3.33 IV retinol
1 RE = 6 flg beta-carotene

Since pure crystalline vitamin A, which is termed retinol alcohol, is now available, the vitamin A activity in foods is now widely expressed and measured using retinol equivalents (RE) rather than the international units (IU) previously used. One IU of vitamin A is equivalent to 0.31 flg retinol.

Humans obtain vitamin A in food either as preformed vitamin A (retinol) or as carotenes which can be converted to retinol in the body. Beta-carotene is the most important in human diets and is better converted to retinol than other carotenes. It has been determined that six molecules of beta-carotene are needed to produce one molecule of retinol; thus it takes 6 flg of carotene to make 1 flg of retinol, or 1 RE.

Dietary Sources

Vitamin A itself is found only in animal products; the main sources are butter, eggs, milk, meat (especially liver) and some fish. However, most people in developing countries rely mainly on beta-carotene for their supply of vitamin A. Carotene is contained in many plant foods. Dark green leaves such as those of amaranth, spinach, sweet potato and cassava are much richer sources than paler leaves such as those of cabbage and lettuce. Various pigmented fruits and vegetables, such as mangoes, papayas and tomatoes, contain useful quantities. Carotene is also present in yellow varieties of sweet potatoes and in yellow vegetables such as pumpkins. Carrots are rich sources. Yellow maize is the only cereal that contains carotene. In West Africa much carotene is obtained from red palm oil, which is widely used in cooking. The cultivation of the very valuable oil palm has spread to other tropical regions. In Malaysia it is widely cultivated as a cash crop, but its products are mainly exported rather than consumed locally.

Both carotene and vitamin A withstand ordinary cooking temperatures fairly well. However, a considerable amount of carotene is lost when green leaves and other foods are dried in the sun. Sun-drying is a traditional method of preserving wild leaves and vegetables often used in arid regions. Since serious disease from vitamin A deficiency is common in these areas, it is important that other methods of preservation be established.

Absorption and Utilization

The conversion of beta-carotene into vitamin A takes place in the walls of the intestines. Even the most efficient intestine can absorb and convert only a portion of the beta-carotene in the diet; therefore 6 mg of beta carotene in food is equivalent to about 1 mg of retinol. If no animal products are consumed and the body must rely entirely on carotene for its vitamin A, consumption of carotene must be great enough to achieve the required vitamin A level.

Carotene is poorly utilized when the diet has a low fat content, and diets deficient in vitamin A are often deficient in fat. Intestinal diseases such as dysentery, coeliac disease and sprue limit the absorption of vitamin A and the conversion of carotene. Malabsorption syndromes and infections with common intestinal parasites such as roundworm, which are prevalent in the tropics, may also reduce the ability of the body to convert carotene into vitamin A.

Bile salts are essential for the absorption of vitamin A and carotene, so persons with obstruction of the bile duct are likely to become deficient in vitamin A. Even in ideal circumstances, infants and young children do not convert carotene to vitamin A as readily as adults do.

The liver acts as the main store of vitamin A in the human and most other vertebrates, which is why fish-liver oils have a high content of this vitamin. Retinol is transported from the liver to other sites in the body by a specific carrier protein called retinol binding protein (RBP). Protein deficiency may influence vitamin A status by reducing the synthesis of RBP.

Storage in the Body

The storage of vitamin A in the liver is important, for in many tropical diets foods containing vitamin A and carotene are available seasonally. If these foods are eaten in fairly large quantities when available (usually during the wet season), a store can be built up which will help tide the person over the dry season, or at least part of it. The short mango season provides an excellent opportunity for youngsters, who may happily spend their leisure hours foraging for this fruit, to replenish the vitamin A stored in the liver.

Toxicity

If taken in excess, vitamin A has undesirable toxic effects. The most marked toxic effect is an irregular thickening of some long bones, usually accompanied by headache, vomiting, liver enlargement, skin changes and hair loss. Cases of vitamin A toxicity from dietary sources are rare, but toxicity can be a serious problem with supplemental doses of vitamin A. A high risk of birth defects is associated with supplements given before or during pregnancy.

Human Requirements

The intake recommended by FAO and the World Health Organization (WHO) is 750 flg of retinol per day for adults; lactating mothers need 50 per cent more, and children and infants less. It should be noted that these figures are based upon mixed diets containing both vitamin A and carotene. When the diet is entirely of vegetable origin, larger amounts of carotene are suggested, because the conversion from carotene to retinol is not very efficient.

Deficiency

Deficiency results in pathological drying of the eye, leading to xerophthalmia and sometimes keratomalacia and blindness. Other epithelial tissues may be affected; in the skin, follicular keratosis may be the result.

Thiamine (Vitamin B1)

During the 1890s in Java, Indonesia, Christiaan Eijkman of the Netherlands noticed that when his chickens were fed on the same diet as that normally consumed by his beriberi patients, they developed weakness in their legs and other signs somewhat similar to those of beriberi. The diet of the beriberi patients consisted mainly of highly milled and refined rice (known as polished rice). When Eijkman changed the diet of the chickens to whole-grain rice, they began to recover. He showed that there was a substance in the outer layers and germ of the rice grain that protected the chickens from the disease.

Researchers continued to work on isolating the cause of the different effectsof diets of polished and whole-grain rice, but despite many attempts it was not until 1926 that vitamin B, was finally isolated in crystalline form. It was synthesized ten years later, and now the term thiamine is used, rather than vitamin B1.

Properties

Thiamine is one of the most unstable vitamins. It has a rather loosely bound structure and decomposes readily in an alkaline medium. Thiamine is highly soluble in water. It resists temperatures of up to 100°C,but it tends to be destroyed if heated further (e.g. if fried in a hot pan or cooked under pressure).

Much research has been carried out on the physiological effects and biochemical properties of thiamine. It has been shown that thiamine has a very important role in carbohydrate metabolism in humans. It is utilized in the complicated mechanism of the breakdown, or oxidation, of carbohydrate and the metabolism of pyruvic acid.

The energy used by the nervous system is derived entirely from carbohydrate, and a deficiency of thiamine blocks the final utilization of carbohydrate, leading to a shortage of energy and lesions of the nervous tissues and brain. Because thiamine is involved in carbohydrate metabolism, a person whose main supply of energy comes from carbohydrates is more likely to develop signs of thiamine deficiency if his or her food intake is decreased. For this reason, thiamine requirements are sometimes expressed in relation to intake of carbohydrate.

Thiamine has been synthesized in pure form and is now measured in milligrams.

Dietary Sources

Thiamine is widely distributed in foods of both vegetable and animal origin. The richest sources are cereal grains and pulses. Green vegetables, fish, meat, fruit and milk all contain useful quantities. In seeds such as cereals, the thiamine is present mainly in the germ and in the outer coats; thus much can be lost during milling. Bran of rice, wheat and other cereals tends to be naturally rich in thiamine. Yeasts are also rich sources. Root crops are poor sources. Cassava, for example, contains only about the same low quantity as polished, highly milled rice. It is surprising that beriberi is not common among the many people in Africa, Asia and Latin America whose staple food is cassava.

Because it is very soluble in water, thiamine is liable to be lost from food that is washed too thoroughly or cooked in excess water that is afterwards discarded. For people on a rice diet, it is especially important to prepare rice with just the amount of water that will be absorbed in cooking, or to use water that is left over in soups or stews, for this water will contain thiamine and other nutrients.

Cereals and pulses maintain their thiamine for a year or more if they are stored well, but if they are attacked by bacteria, insects or moulds the content of thiamine gradually diminishes.

Absorption and Storage in the Body

Thiamine is easily absorbed from the intestinal tract, but little is stored in the body. Experimental evidence indicates that humans can store only enough for about six weeks. The liver, heart and brain have a higher concentration than the muscles and other organs. A person with a high intake of thiamine soon begins to excrete increased quantities in the urine. The total amount in the body is about 25 mg.

Human Requirements

A daily intake of 1 mg of thiamine is sufficient for a moderately active man and 0.8 mg for a moderately active woman. Pregnant and lactating women may need more. FAO and WHO recommend an intake of 0.4 mg per 1000 kcal for most persons.

Deficiency

Deficiency of thiamine leads to the disease beriberi, which in advanced forms produces paralysis of the limbs. In alcoholics thiamine deficiency leads to a condition termed Wernicke-Korsakoff syndrome.

Riboflavin (Vitamin B2)

Early work on the properties of vitamins in' yeast and other foodstuffs showed that antineuritic factors were destroyed by excessive heat, but that a growth-promoting factor was not destroyed in this way. This factor, riboflavin, was later isolated from the heat-resistant portion. It was synthesized in 1935.

Properties

Riboflavin is a yellow crystalline substance. It is much less soluble in water and more heat resistant than thiamine. The vitamin is sensitive to sunlight, so milk, for example, if left exposed may lose considerable quantities of riboflavin. Riboflavin acts as a coenzyme involved with tissue oxidation. It is measured in milligrams.

Dietary Sources

The richest sources of riboflavin are milk and its non-fat products. Green vegetables, meat (especially liver), fish and eggs contain useful quantities.

However, the main sources in most Asian, African and Latin American diets, which do not contain much of the products, are usually cereal grains and pulses. As with thiamine, the quantity of riboflavin present is much reduced by milling. Starchy foods such as cassava, plantains, yams and sweet potatoes are poor sources.

Human Requirements

Approximately 1.5 mg of riboflavin per day is an ample amount for an average adult, but rather more may be desirable during pregnancy and lactation. The FAO/WHO requirement is 0.55 mg per 1000 kcal in the diet.

Deficiency

Inhumans a deficiency of riboflavin is termed ariboflavinosis. It may be characterized by painful cracking of the lips (cheilosis) and at the comers of the mouth (angular stomatitis). Ariboflavinosis is common in most countries but is not life threatening.

Niacin (Nicotinic Acid, Nicotinamide, Vitamin PP)

As the history of thiamine is linked with the disease beriberi, so the history of niacin is closely linked with the disease pellagra. beriberi is associated with the East and a rice diet, and pellagra with the West and a maize diet.

Pellagra was first attributed to a poor diet over 200 years ago by the Spanish physician Gaspar Casal. At first, it was believed that pellagra might be caused by a protein deficiency, because the disease could be cured by some diets rich in protein. Later it was shown that a liver extract almost devoid of protein could cure pellagra.

J. Goldberger, in 1926 in the United States, demonstrated that yeast extract contained a pellagra-preventing (PP) non-protein substance. In 1937 niacinamide or nicotinamide (nicotinic acid amide) was isolated, and this was found to cure a pellagra-like disease of dogs known as black tongue.

Because pellagra was found mainly in those whose staple diet was maize, it was assumed that maize was particularly poor in niacin. It has since been shown that white bread contains much less niacin than maize. However, the niacin in maize is not fully available because it is in a bound form.

The discovery that the amino acid tryptophan prevents pellagra in experimental animals, just as niacin does, complicated the picture until it was shown that tryptophan is converted to niacin in the human body. This work vindicated and explained the early theories that protein could prevent pellagra. The fact that zein, the main protein in maize, is very deficient in the amino acid tryptophan further explains the relationship between maize and pellagra. It has also been shown that a high intake of leucine, as occurs with diets based on sorghum, interferes with tryptophan and niacin metabolism and may cause pellagra.

Properties

Niacin, a derivative of pyridine, is a white crystalline substance, soluble in water and extremely stable. It has been synthesized. The main role of niacin in the body is in tissue oxidation. The vitamin occurs in two forms, nicotinic acid and nicotinamide (niacinamide). Niacin is measured in milligrams.

Dietary Sources

Niacin is widely distributed in foods of both animal and vegetable origin. Particularly good sources are meat (especially liver), groundnuts and cereal bran or germ. As for other B vitamins, the main source of supply tends to be the staple food. whole-grain or lightly milled cereals, although not rich in niacin, contain much more than highly milled cereal grains.

Starchy roots, plantains and milk are poor sources. Beans, peas and other pulses contain amounts similar to those in most cereals.

Although the niacin in maize does not seem to be fully utilizable, treatment of maize with alkalis such as lime water, which is a traditional method of processing in Mexico and elsewhere, makes the niacin much more available.

Cooking, preservation and storage of food cause little loss of niacin.

Human Requirements

An adequate quantity for any person is 20 mg per day. Niacin requirements are affected by the amount of tryptophan containing protein consumed and also by the staple diet (i.e., whether it is maize-based or not). The FAO/WHO requirement is 6.6 mg per 1000 kcal in the diet.

Deficiency

A deficiency of niacin leads to pellagra, the 'disease of the three Ds': dermatitis, diarrhoea and dementia. Initially manifested as skin trouble, pellagra, if untreated, can continue for many years, growing steadily worse.

Vitamin B12 (Cyanocobalamin)

Pernicious anaemia, so named because it invariably used to be fatal, was known for many years before its cause 'was determined. In 1926 it was found that patients improved if they ate raw liver.

This finding led to the preparation of liver extracts, which controlled the disease when given by injection. In 1948 scientists isolated from liver a substance they called vitamin B12.When given in very small quantities by injection, this substance was effective in the treatment of pernicious anaemia.

Properties

Vitamin B12 is a red crystalline substance containing the metal cobalt. It is necessary for the production of healthy red blood cells. A small addition of vitamin B12or of foods rich in this substance to the diet of experimental animals results in increased growth. It is measured in micrograms.

Dietary Sources

Vitamin B12 is present only in foods of animal origin. It can also be synthesized by many bacteria. Herbivorous animals such as cattle get their vitamin B12from the action of bacteria on vegetable matter in their rumen. Humans apparently do not obtain vitamin B12 by bacterial action in their digestive tracts. However, fermented vegetable products may provide vitamin B12 in human diets.

Human Requirements

The human daily requirement of this vitamin is quite small, probably around 3 flg for adults. Diets containing smaller amounts do not seem to lead to disease.

Deficiency

Pernicious anaemia is not caused by a dietary deficiency of vitamin B12 but by an inability of the subject to utilize the vitamin B12 in the diet because of a lack of an intrinsic factor in gastric secretions. It may be that an autoimmune reaction limits absorption of vitamin B12. In pernicious anaemia the red blood cells are macrocytic (larger than normal) and the bone marrow contains many abnormal cells called megaloblasts. This macrocytic or megaloblastic anemia is accompanied by a lack of hydrochloric acid in the stomach (achlorhydria). Later, serious changes take place in the spinal cord, leading to progressive neurological symptoms. If left untreated, the patient dies.

Treatment consists of injection of large doses of vitamin B12 When the blood characteristics have returned to normal, the patient can usually be maintained in good health if given one injection of 250 mg of vitamin B12 every two to four weeks.

Vitamin B12 will also cure the anemia accompanying the disease sprue. This is a tropical condition in which the absorption of vitamin B12,folic acid and other nutrients is impaired.

The tapeworm *Diphyllobothrium latum,* acquired from eating raw or undercooked fish, lives in the intestines and has a propensity for removing vitamin B12 from the food of its host. This results in the development in humans of a megaloblastic anemia which can be cured by injection of vitamin B12 and treatment to rid the patient of the tapeworm.

Some medicines interfere with absorption of vitamin B12.

Except in the deficiency of vitamin B12 is likely to occur only in those on a vegetarian diet. Deficiency causes macrocytic anaemia and may produce neurological symptoms; however, even though strict vegetarians get very little vitamin B12 in their diet, it appears that macrocytic anemia due to vitamin B12 deficiency is not prevalent and is not a major public health problem.

Vitamin B 17

Vitamin B 17 belongs to the category of Vitamin B complex. Scientists identified the component Amygdalin, which is responsible for raising the count of white blood cells. The vitamin is found abundantly in the seeds of plants of the prunasin family like apricots and apples. Considered as a nitriloside, a natural cyanide containing substance, its extract Laetrile is a popular supplement. Its anti-cancerous properties aside, Vitamin B17, especially if derived from natural food sources instead of supplements, can bring in a bevy of health benefits. They include:

Regulating Hypertension: Vitamin B17 can help regulate hypertension issues due to the formation of thiocyanate, instrumental in lowering high blood pressure.

Boosts the Immune System: Vitamin B17 is also known to work wonders for the immune system. The biggest benefit of the vitamin to be its potential to increase white blood cells, which improve immunity.

Great Antioxidant: Some experts also claim the ability of the vitamin to associate with other powerful antioxidants like vitamin A, C and E to break down and eradicate toxic cells from our body, thus aiding a natural detox process and promoting overall health.

Pain Reliever: Vitamin B17 also works as an effective pain reliever.

Dietary Sources

Here is a list of Vitamin B17 sources that should come handy to you, if you are looking to maximise on the benefits of this nutrient:

1. Seeds

Many seeds and kernels of various fruits are rich in the vitamin, apricot kernels and seeds being on top of the chart. Other seeds loaded with goodness of vitamin B17 are apple seeds, plum seeds and pear seeds. Tiny seeds of berries, grapes, strawberries and raspberries. Flax seeds, squash seeds, millet seeds and buckwheat seeds are also found to contain this vitamin in adequate amounts.

2. Berries

Raspberries, elderberries, strawberries, blueberries, blackberries and wild berries contain the vitamin in pretty abundant quantities.

3. Nuts

Did you know that the bitter variant of almond was used in abundance traditionally by the Chinese, Egyptians and Pueblo Indians in around 1802, it was identified that distilling the water from bitter almonds releases hydrocyanic acid, which could be purified to form Amygdalin. Macedemia nuts and cashew nuts follow next after bitter almonds in terms of vitamin B17 content.

4. Grains and Millets

Load up on sorghum, buckwheat, barley and millet from your kitchen pantry to optimise on the nutritional benefit of the vitamin.

5. Eucalyptus Leaves

Leaves of Eucalyptus are found to contain moderate amounts of vitamin B17. Even spinach leaves are said to have traces of the vitamin.

6. Sprouts

Bamboo sprouts or bamboo shoots boast of a high content of the vitamin, followed by the sprouts of alfalfa, fava beans and mung sprouts. Whole green gram sprouts also contain the vitamin but in very moderate amounts.

Other Dietary Sources;

Foods Rich in Vitamin B17 , native non-hybridized Apples; mostly crab Apples, native non-hybridized wild fruit; wild fruit; Alfalfa Sprouts, Almonds, Apple Seeds, Apricot Kernels,

Avocado Seed, Bamboo Shoots, Barley, Beet Tops, Bitter Almond, Blackberries, Boysenberries, Brewers Yeast, Butter Beans, Brown Rice, Buckwheat, Cashew Nuts, Cherry Kernels, Chia Seeds, Cranberries, Currants, Elderberry, Eucalyptus Leaves, Fava Beans, Flax Seeds, Garbanzo Beans, Gooseberries, Grasses, Huckleberries, Lentils, Lima Beans, Flax Meal, Loganberries, Macadamia Nuts, Milkweed, Millet, Millet Seeds, Mung Beans Sprouts, Nuts, Oat Groats, Passion Fruit, Peach Kernels, Pear Seeds, Quince, Raspberries, Rye Seeds, Sesame Seeds, Sorghum Spelt , Strawberries, Sweet Potato, Tamarind, Yams, and other seeds of plants of the prunasin family.

It's time to make sure you eat a little of these on a constant basis, in reasonable amounts, for cancer and other malignancy prevention and boosting your immunity system.

Folic Acid or Folates

In 1929 Lucy Wills first described a macrocytic anemia (an anemia in which the red cells are abnormally large) commonly found among pregnant women in developing countries. This condition responded to certain yeast preparations even though it did not respond to iron or any known vitamin. The substance present in the yeast extract that cured the macrocytic anemia was at first called 'Wills factor'. In 1946 a substance called folic acid, which had been isolated from spinach leaves, was found to have the same effect.

Properties

Folic acid is the group name (also termed folates or folacin) given to a number of yellow crystalline compounds related to pteroglutamic acid. Folic acid is involved in amino acid metabolism. The folic acid in foodstuffs is easily destroyed by cooking. It is measured in milligrams.

Dietary Sources

The richest sources are dark green leaves, liver and kidney. Other vegetables and meats contain smaller amounts.

Human Requirements

The recommended daily intake for adults has been set at 400 flg in the United States.

Deficiency

Folate deficiency is most commonly due to poor diets, but it may result from malabsorption. It can be induced by medicines such as those used in treatment of epilepsy. A deficiency leads to the development of macrocytic anemia. Anemia resulting from folate deficiency is the second most common type of nutritional anemia, after iron deficiency.

Folic acid deficiency during pregnancy has been found to cause neural tube defects in newborn babies. The role of folic acid in prevention of ischaemic heart disease has also recently received increased attention.

The main therapeutic use of folic acid is in the treatment of nutritional macrocytic or megaloblastic anemias of pregnancy and infancy and for the prevention of neural tube defects. A dose of 5 to 10 mg daily is recommended for an adult.

Although administration of folic acid will improve the blood picture of persons with pernicious anemia, the nervous system symptoms will neither be prevented nor improved by it. For this reason, folic acid should never be used in the treatment of pernicious anemia, except in conjunction with vitamin B12.

Vitamin C (Aascorbic Acid)

The discovery of vitamin C is associated with scurvy, which was first recorded by seafarers who made prolonged journeys.

In 1497 Vasco da Gama described scurvy among the crew of his historical voyage from Europe around the southern tip of Africa to India; more than half the crew died of the disease.

It gradually became apparent that scurvy occurred only in persons who ate no fresh food. It was in 1747, James Lind of Scotland demonstrated that scurvy could be prevented or cured by the consumption of citrus fruit. This finding led to the introduction of fresh food, especially citrus products, to the rations of seafarers. Subsequently scurvy became much less common.

In the nineteenth century, however, scurvy began to occur among infants receiving the newly introduced preserved milk instead of breastmilk or fresh cows' milk. The preserved milk contained adequate carbohydrate, fat, protein and minerals, but the heat used in its processing destroyed the vitamin C, so the infants got scurvy.

Later vitamin C was found to be ascorbic acid, which had already been identified.

Properties

Ascorbic acid is a white crystalline substance that is highly soluble in water. It tends to be easily oxidized. It is not affected by light, but it is destroyed by excessive heat, especially when in an alkaline solution. It is a powerful reducing agent and antioxidant and can therefore reduce the harmful action of free radicals. It is also important in enhancing the absorption of the non-haem iron in foods of vegetable origin.

Ascorbic acid is necessary for the proper formation and maintenance of intercellular material, particularly collagen. In simple terms, it is essential for producing part of the substance that binds cells together, as cement binds bricks together.

In a person suffering from ascorbic acid deficiency, the endothelial cells of the capillaries lack normal solidification. They are therefore fragile, and haemorrhages take place. Similarly, the dentine of the teeth and the osteoid tissue of the bone are improperly formed. This cell-binding property also explains the poor scar formation and slow healing of wounds manifest in persons deficient in ascorbic acid.

It is a common belief, claimed also by some scientists, that very large doses of vitamin C both prevent and reduce symptoms of the common cold (coryza).This claim has not been verified. One large study did suggest a modest reduction in the severity of cold symptoms in those taking vitamin C medicinally, but the vitamin Did not prevent colds from occurring. It is not advisable to take very large doses of medicinal vitamin C for long periods of time.

Dietary Sources

The main sources of vitamin C in most diets are fruits, vegetables and various leaves. In pastoral tribes milk is often the main source. Plantains and bananas are the only common staple foods containing fair quantities of vitamin C. Dark green leaves such as amaranth and spinach contain far more than pale leaves such as cabbage and lettuce. Root vegetables and potatoes contain small but useful quantities. Young maize provides some ascorbic acid, as do sprouted cereals and pulses. Animal products such as meat, fish, milk and eggs contain small quantities.

As vitamin C is easily destroyed by heat, prolonged cooking of any food may destroy much of the vitamin C present.

Ascorbic acid is measured in milligrams of the pure vitamin.

Human Requirements

Opinions regarding human requirements differ widely. It seems clear that as much as 75 mg per day is necessary if the body is to remain fully saturated with vitamin C. However, individuals appear to remain healthy on intakes as low as 10 mg per day. A recommendation of 25 mg for an adult, 30 mg for adolescents, 35 mg during pregnancy and 45 mg during lactation seems to be a reasonable compromise.

Deficiency

Scurvy and the other clinical manifestations of vitamin C deficiency are described in Chapter 19. Scurvy is not now a prevalent disease. Outbreaks have occurred in famine areas and recently in several refugee camps in Africa. In its early stages vitamin C deficiency may lead to bleeding gums and slow healing of wounds.

Vitamin D

Vitamin D is associated with prevention of the disease rickets and its adult counterpart osteomalacia (softening of the bones). Rickets was for many years suspected to be a nutritional deficiency disease, and in certain parts of the world cod-liver oil was used in its treatment. However, in 1919 Sir Edward Mellanby, using puppies, demonstrated conclusively that the disease was indeed of nutritional origin and that it responded to vitamin D in cod-liver oil. Later it was proved that action of sunlight on the skin leads to the production of the vitamin D used by humans.

Properties

A number of compounds, all sterols closely related to cholesterol, possess antirachitic properties. It was found that certain sterols that did not have these properties became antirachitic when acted upon by ultraviolet light. The two important activated sterols are vitamin D2 (ergocalciferol) and vitamin D3 (cholecalciferol).

In human beings, when the skin is exposed to the ultraviolet rays of sunlight, a sterol compound is activated to form vitamin D, which is then available to the body and which has exactly the same function as vitamin D taken in the diet. Dietary vitamin D is only absorbed from the gut in the presence of bile.

The function of vitamin D in the body is to allow the proper absorption of calcium. Vitamin D formed in the skin or absorbed from food acts like a hormone in influencing calcium metabolism. Rickets and osteomalacia, though diseases in which calcium is deficient in certain tissues, are caused not by calcium deficiency in the diet but by a lack of vitamin D which would allow proper utilization of the calcium in the diet.

Vitamin D is often expressed in international units; 1 IV is equivalent to 0.025 flg of vitamin D3.

Dietary Sources

Vitamin D occurs naturally only in the fat in certain animal products. Eggs, cheese, milk and butter are good sources in normal diets. Meat and fish contribute small quantities. Fish-liver oils are very rich. Cereals, vegetables and fruit contain no vitamin D.

Storage in the Body

The body has a considerable capacity to store vitamin D in fatty tissue and in the liver. An adequate store is important in a pregnant woman, to avoid predisposition to rickets in the child.

Human Requirements

It is not possible to define human dietary requirements, because the vitamin is obtained both by eating foods containing vitamin

D and by the action of sunlight on the skin. There is no need for adults to have any vitamin D in their diets, provided they are adequately exposed to sunlight, and many children in Asia, Latin America and Africa survive in good health on a diet almost completely devoid of vitamin D. It has been shown that fish-liver oil containing 400 IV (10 ug) of vitamin D will prevent the occurrence of rickets in infants or children not exposed to sunlight. This amount seems to be a safe allowance.

Deficiency

Rickets and osteomalacia, two diseases resulting from a deficiency of vitamin D, are described in Chapter 18. As vitamin. D is produced in humans by the action of the sun on the skin, deficiency is not common in tropical countries, although synthesis of vitamin D may possibly be reduced in darkly pigmented skin. Rickets and osteomalacia are seen sporadically but are more common in areas where tradition or religion keeps women and children indoors. Many cases have been reported from Yemen and Ethiopia. The conditions are manifested mainly by skeletal changes.

Toxicity

Like other fat-soluble vitamins, vitamin D taken in excess in the diet is not well excreted. Consumption of large doses, which has most commonly resulted from overdosing of children with fish-liver oil preparations, can lead to toxicity. Overdosing may lead to hypercalcaemia, diagnosed from high levels of calcium in the blood. Toxicity usually begins with loss of appetite and weight, which may be followed by mental disorientation and finally by kidney failure. Fatalities have been recorded.

Other Vitamins

The two fat-soluble vitamins (A and D) and the six water-soluble vitamins (thiamine, riboflavin, niacin, vitamin B12 folates and vitamin C) . have been described in some detail because these are the vitamins most likely to be deficient and to be of public health importance in non industrialized countries. Five other vitamins, although vital to human health, are not very commonly deficient in human diets and so are of less public health importance. These are vitamin B 5, pantothenic acid, vitamin E and vitamin K.

Vitamin B6 (Pyridoxine)

Vitamin B6is a water-soluble vitamin widely present in foods of both animal and vegetable origin. It is important as a coenzyme in many metabolic processes. Primary dietary deficiency is extremely rare, but vitamin B6 deficiency became common in tuberculosis patients treated with the drug isoniazid. The patients developed neurological signs and sometimes also anemia and dermatosis. Now it is common to provide 10 mg of vitamin B6 by mouth daily to those receiving large doses of isoniazid. Vitamin B6 is relatively expensive, however, and the routine administration of vitamin B6 to patients receiving isoniazid increases the cost of treatment of tuberculosis.

Biotin

Biotin is another water-soluble vitamin of the B complex group. It is found widely in food, and deficiency in humans is extremely rare. The vitamin is very important, however, in physiological and biochemical metabolic processes. Avidin in uncooked egg white prevents absorption of biotin in animals and humans. Rats fed egg white as their only source of protein become thin and wasted and develop neuropathies and dermatitis. Biotin deficiency has been reported in a very few cases, in people consuming mainly egg white and in a few intravenously-fed patients with some special forms of malabsorption.

Pantothenic Acid

Pantothenic acid, a water-soluble vitamin, is present in adequate amounts in almost all human diets. It has important biochemical functions in various enzyme reactions, but deficiency in humans is very rare. A neurological condition described as burning feet syndrome, reported in prisoners of war held by the Japanese between 1942 and 1945, was ascribed to a deficiency of this vitamin.

Vitamin E (Tocopherol)

Vitamin E, a fat-soluble vitamin, is obtained by humans mainly from vegetable oils and whole-grain cereals. It has been termed the 'anti-sterility' or 'sex vitamin' because rats fed on tocopherol-deficient diets cannot reproduce: males develop abnormalities in the testicles and females abort spontaneously.

Because of its relationship to fertility and to many conditions in animals, vitamin E is widely self-prescribed and is not uncommonly recommended by physicians for a variety of human ills. However, true deficiency is probably rare; it occurs mainly in association with severe malabsorption states (when fat is poorly absorbed), in genetic anaemias [including glucose-6-phosphatase dehydrogenase (G-6PD) deficiency] and occasionally in very low-weight babies.

Vitamin E (like vitamin C) is an antioxidant, and because of its ability to limit oxidation and to deal with damaging free radicals it is sometimes recommended as a possible preventive for both arteriosclerosis and cancer. Its presence in oils helps prevent the oxidation of unsaturated fatty acids.

Vitamin K

Vitamin K has been termed the 'coagulation vitamin' because of its relationship to prothrombin and blood coagulation, and because it is successfully used to treat a bleeding condition of newborn infants (haemorrhagic disease of the newborn). Humans obtain some vitamin K from food, and some is also made by bacteria in the intestines. Newborn infants have a gut free of organisms, so they do not get vitamin K from bacterial synthesis. It is now believed that intravenously fed or starved patients receiving broad-spectrum antibiotics that kill gut bacteria may bleed because of vitamin K deficiency. In many hospitals vitamin K is given routinely to newborn infants to prevent haemorrhagic disease.

4
Digestion and Absorption

The major components of the diet are starches, sugars, fats, and proteins. These have to be hydrolyzed to their constituent smaller molecules for absorption and metabolism. Starches and sugars are absorbed as monosaccharides, fats as free fatty acids and glycerol (plus a small amount of intact triacylglycerol), and proteins as their constituent amino acids and small peptides.

The fat-soluble vitamins (A, D, E, and K) are absorbed dissolved in dietary lipids; there are active transport systems in the small intestinal mucosa for the absorp- tion of the water-soluble vitamins. The absorption of vitamin B12 requires a specific binding protein that is secreted in the gastric juice in order to bind to the mucosal transport system.

Minerals generally enter the intestinal mucosal cells by carrier-mediated diffusion and are accumulated intracellularly by binding to specific binding proteins. They are then transferred into the bloodstream by active transport mechanisms at the serosal side of the epithelial cells, usually onto plasma-binding proteins.

The Gastrointestinal Tract

The major functions of each region of gastrointestinal tract are discussed below.

Mouth

Hydrolysis of a small amount of starch catalyzed by amylase, secreted by the salivary glands. Hydrolysis of a small amount of fat, catalyzed by lingual lipase, secreted by the tongue. Absorption of small amounts of vitamin C.

Stomach

Denaturation of dietary proteins (Section 4.4.2.3) and the release of vitamin B12, iron, and other minerals from protein binding, for which gastric acid is important. Hydrolysis of protein catalyzed by pepsin. Hydrolysis of fat catalyzed by lipase. Secretion of intrinsic factor for the absorption of vitamin B12.

Small intestine (duodenum, jejunum, and ileum)

Hydrolysis of starch catalyzed by amylase secreted by the pancreas. Hydrolysis of disaccharides within the brush border of the intestinal mucosa.

Hydrolysis of fat catalyzed by lipase, phospholipase, and esterase secreted by the pancreas. Hydrolysis of protein catalyzed by a variety of exo- and endopeptidases secreted by the pancreas and small-intestinal mucosa.

Hydrolysis of di- and tripeptides within the brush border of the intestinal mucosa. Absorption of the products of digestion. Absorption of water (failure of water absorption, as in diarrhea, can lead to serious dehydration).

Large intestine (cecum and colon)

Bacterial metabolism of undigested carbohydrates, proteins, and shed intestinal mucosal cells. Absorption of some of the products of bacterial metabolism. Absorption of water.

Rectum

Storage of undigested gut contents prior to evacuation as feces.

Throughout the gastrointestinal tract, and especially in the small intestine, the surface area of the mucosa is considerably greater than would appear from its superficial appearance. The intestinal mucosa is folded into the lumen. The surface of these folds is covered with villi, fingerlike projections into the lumen, some 0.5–1.5 mm long. There are some 20–40 villi/mm2, giving a total absorptive surface area of some 300 m2 in the small intestine.

Each villus has both blood capillaries, which drain into the hepatic portal vein, and a lacteal, which drains into the lymphatic system. Water-soluble products of digestion (carbohydrates and amino acids) are absorbed into the blood capillaries, and the liver has a major role in controlling the availability of the products of carbohydrate and protein digestion to other tissues in the body. Lipids are absorbed into the lacteals; the lymphatic system joins the bloodstream at the thoracic duct; and extrahepatic tissues are exposed to the products of lipid digestion uncontrolled by the liver, which functions to clear the remnants from the circulation.

There is rapid turnover of the cells of the intestinal mucosa; epithelial cells proliferate in the crypts, alongside the cells that secrete digestive enzymes and mucus, and migrate to the tip of the villus, where they are shed into the lumen. The average life of an intestinal mucosal epithelial cell is about 48 h. This rapid turnover of epithelial cells is important in controlling the absorption of iron and possibly other minerals.

The rapid turnover of intestinal mucosal cells is also important for protection against the digestive enzymes secreted into the lumen. Further protection is afforded by the secretion of mucus, a solution of mucin and other proteins that are resistant to enzymic hydrolysis, which coats the intestinal mucosa. The secretion of intestinal mucus explains a considerable part of an adult's continuing requirement for dietary protein .

Digestion and Absorption of Carbohydrates

Carbohydrates are compounds of carbon, hydrogen, and oxygen in the ratio Cn:H2n:On. The basic unit of the carbohydrates is the sugar molecule or monosaccharide. Note that sugar is used here in a chemical sense and includes a variety of simple carbohydrates, which are collectively known as sugars. Ordinary table sugar (cane sugar or beet sugar) is correctly known as sucrose; it is a disaccharide . It is only one of a number of different sugars found in the diet.

Dietary carbohydrates can be considered in two main groups: sugars and polysaccharides; the polysaccharides can be further subdivided into starches and nonstarch polysaccharides . The simplest type of sugar is a monosaccharide; a single sugar unit . Monosaccharides consist of between three and seven carbon atoms and the corresponding number of hydrogen and oxygen atoms. A few larger monosaccharides also occur, although they are not important in nutrition and metabolism.

Disaccharides are formed by condensation between two monosaccharides to form a glycoside bond. The reverse reaction, cleavage of the glycoside bond to release the individual monosaccharides, is a hydrolysis.

Oligosaccharides consist of three or four monosaccharide units (trisaccharides and tetrasaccharides), and occasionally more, linked by glycoside bonds. Most are not digested, but are fermented by intestinal bacteria, yielding short-chain fatty acids that provide a metabolic fuel to intestinal mucosal cells, and may be protective against colorectal cancer . The oligosaccharides also make a significant contribution to the production of intestinal gas.

Nutritionally, it is useful to consider sugars (both monosaccharides and disaccharides) in two groups:

Intrinsic sugars that are contained within plant cell walls in foods.

Sugars that are in free solution in foods, and therefore provide a substrate for oral bacteria, leading to the formation of dental plaque and caries. These are known as extrinsic sugars; it is considered desirable to reduce the consumption of extrinsic sugars , both because of their role in dental decay and also because of the ease with which excessive amounts of sweet foods can be consumed, thus leading to obesity.

A complication in the classification of sugars as intrinsic (which are considered desirable in the diet) and extrinsic (which are considered undesirable in the diet) is that lactose is in free solution in milk, and hence is an extrinsic sugar. However, lactose is not a cause of dental decay, and milk is an important source of calcium , protein , and vitamin B2 . It is not considered desirable to reduce intakes of milk, which is the only significant source of lactose, and extrinsic sugars are further subdivided into milk sugar and nonmilk extrinsic sugars.

Polysaccharides are polymers of many hundreds of monosaccharide units, again linked by glycoside bonds. The most important are starch and glycogen, both of which are polymers of glucose. There are a number of other polysaccharides, composed of other monosaccharides, or of glucose units linked differently from the linkages in starch and glycogen. Collectively these are known as nonstarch polysaccharides. They are generally not digested but have important roles in nutrition . The classes of monosaccharides are named by the number of carbon atoms in the ring, using the Greek names for the numbers, with the ending '-ose' to show that they are sugars. The names of all sugars end in '-ose' are provided, viz., 3-carbon monosaccharides are trioses, 4-carbon monosaccharides are tetroses, 5-carbon monosaccharides are pentoses, 6-carbon monosaccharides are hexoses, and 7-carbon monosaccharides are heptoses.

In general, trioses, tetroses, and heptoses are important as intermediate compounds in the metabolism of pentoses and hexoses. Hexoses are the nutritionally important sugars.

The pentoses and hexoses can exist as either straight-chain compounds or can form heterocyclic rings. By convention, the ring of sugars is drawn with the bonds of one side thicker than the other. This is to show that the rings are planar and can be considered to lie at right angles to the plane of the paper. The boldly drawn part of the molecule comes forward out of the paper, and the lightly drawn part goes behind the paper. The hydroxyl groups lie above or below the plane of the ring in the plane of the paper. Each carbon has a hydrogen atom attached as well as a hydroxyl group; this is generally omitted when the structures are drawn as rings.

The nutritionally important hexoses are glucose, galactose, and fructose. Glucose and galactose differ from each other only in the arrangement of one hydroxyl group above or below the plane of the ring. Fructose differs from glucose and galactose in that it has a C=O (keto) group at carbon 2, while the other two have an H–C=O (aldehyde) group at carbon 1.

There are two important pentose sugars, ribose and deoxyribose. Deoxyribose is unusual, in that it has lost one of its hydroxyl groups. The main role of ribose and deoxyribose is in the nucleotides and the nucleic acids; ribonucleic acid

(RNA) in which the sugar is ribose, and DNA, in which the sugar is deoxyribose . Although pentoses do occur in the diet, they are also readily synthesized from glucose . Sugar alcohols (or polyols) are formed by the reduction of the aldehyde group of a monosaccharide to a hydroxyl (–OH) group. Quantitatively, the most important is sorbitol, formed by the reduction of glucose. It is poorly absorbed from the intestinal tract, so that it has very much less effect on blood glucose than other carbohydrates. Because of this, it is widely used in preparation of foods suitable for use by diabetics, since it tastes sweet, and can replace sucrose and other sugars in food manufacture. However, it is metabolized as a metabolic fuel, although because of its poor absorption, it has an energy yield approximately half that of glucose, so that it is not suitable for the replacement of sugar in weight-reducing diets.

Sugar alcohols are poor substrates for metabolism by the plaque-forming bacteria that are associated with dental caries and are used in the manufacture of "tooth-friendly" sweets and chewing gum. There is some evidence that xylitol, the sugar alcohol formed by reduction of the 5-carbon sugar xylose (an isomer of ribose), may have a positive effect in preventing dental caries. The major dietary disaccharides are the following: Sucrose, cane or beet sugar, which is glucosyl-fructose, Lactose, the sugar of milk, which is galactosyl-glucose, Maltose, the sugar originally isolated from malt, and a product of starch digestion,which is glucosyl-glucose, Isomaltose, a product of starch digestion, which is glucosyl-glucose linked 1→6, and Trehalose, found especially in mushrooms, but also as the blood sugar of some insects, which is glucosyl-glucoside. Chemically, the aldehyde group of glucose is a reducing agent. This provides a simple test for glucose in urine (Figure 4.6). Glucose reacts with copper (Cu^{2+}) ions in alkaline solution, reducing them to Cu^{+} oxide and itself being oxidized. The original solution of Cu^{2+} ions has a blue colour; the copper oxide forms a red-brown precipitate. This reaction is not specific for glucose. Other sugars with a free aldehyde group at carbon-1, including vitamin C, and a number of pentose sugars that occur in foods can undergo the same reaction, giving a false-positive result.

While alkaline copper reagents are sometimes used to measure urine glucose in monitoring diabetic control, a test using the enzyme glucose oxidase measures only glucose. Glucose oxidase reduces oxygen to hydrogen peroxide, which, in the presence of catalase, can be reduced to water by oxidation of the colorless compound ABTS to yield a blue color that can readily be measured. High concentrations of vitamin C, as may occur in the urine of people taking supplements of the vitamin, can react with hydrogen peroxide before it oxidizes the colorless precursor or can reduce the dyestuff back to its colorless form. This means that tests using glucose oxidase can yield a false-negative result in the presence of high concentrations of vitamin C.

The term reducing sugars reflects a chemical reaction of the sugars; the ability to reduce a suitable acceptor such as copper ions. It has nothing to do with weight reduction and slimming, although some people erroneously believe that reducing sugars somehow help one to reduce excessive weight. This is not correct, the energy yield from reducing sugars and non-reducing sugars is exactly the same, and excess of either will contribute to obesity.

Starch is a polymer of glucose containing a large but variable number of glucose units. It is thus impossible to quote a relative molecular mass for starch or discuss amounts of starch in terms of moles. It can, however, be hydrolyzed to glucose, and the results expressed as moles of glucose.

The simplest type of starch is amylose, a straight chain of glucose molecules, with glycoside links between carbon-1 of one glucose unit and carbon-4 of the next. Amylopectin has a branched structure, where every thirtieth glucose molecule has glycoside links to three others instead of just two. The branch is formed by linkage between carbon-1 of one glucose unit and carbon-6 of the next glucose unit. Starches are the storage carbohydrates of plants, and the relative amounts of amylose and amylopectin differ in starches from different sources, as indeed does the size of the overall starch molecule. On average, about 20%–25% of dietary starch is amylose and the remaining 75%– 80%, amylopectin.

Glycogen is the storage carbohydrate of mammalian muscle and liver. It is synthesized from glucose in the fed state, and its constituent glucose units are used as a metabolic fuel in the fasting state. Glycogen is a branched polymer with a similar structure to amylopectin, but more highly branched with a 1→6 bond about every tenth glucose. Because of its highly branched structure, glycogen traps a great deal of water in the cell; as glycogen stores are depleted during a period of fasting or reduced food intake, this water is released, leading to a considerable loss of body weight during the early stages of food restriction .

Dietary fibres

There are a number of other polysaccharides in foods. Collectively they are known as non-starch polysaccharides and are the major components of dietary fibre. Non-starch polysaccharides are not digested by human enzymes, although all can be fermented to some extent by intestinal bacteria, and the products of bacterial fermentation may be absorbed and metabolized as metabolic fuels. The major non-starch polysaccharides are; Cellulose, a polymer of glucose in which the configuration of the glycoside bond between the glucose units is in the opposite configuration ($\beta 1 \rightarrow 4$) from that in starch ($\alpha 1 \rightarrow 4$) and cannot be hydrolyzed by human enzymes, Hemicelluloses, branched polymers of pentose (5-carbon) and hexose (6-carbon) sugars, Inulin, a polymer of fructose, which is the storage carbohydrate of Jerusalem artichoke and some other root vegetables, Pectin, a complex polymer of a variety of monosaccharides, including some methylated sugars, Plant gums such as gum arabic, gum tragacanth, acacia, carob, and guar gums; complex polymers of mixed monosaccharides, Mucilages such as alginates, agar, and carrageen; complex polymers of mixed monosaccharides found in seaweeds and other algae.

Cellulose, hemicelluloses, and inulin are insoluble nonstarch polysaccharides, while pectin and the plant gums and mucilages are soluble. The other major constituent of dietary fiber, lignin, is not a carbohydrate at all, but a complex polymer of a variety of aromatic alcohols.

Soluble non-starch polysaccharides increase the viscosity of the intestinal contents and so slow the absorption of the products of digestion. This can be valuable in the treatment of diabetes mellitus and a number of studies have shown that consuming a relatively large amount of soluble non-starch polysaccharide before a meal lowers the postprandial rise of blood glucose, thus enhancing glycemic control. Insoluble non-starch polysaccharides increase the bulk of the intestinal contents, thus aiding peristalsis; they may also adsorb the bile salts and potential carcinogens in the diet, thus reducing their absorption.

Both soluble and insoluble non-starch polysaccharides, as well as oligosaccharides and starch that is resistant to digestion are substrates for bacterial fermentation in the large intestine, yielding short-chain fatty acids (especially butyrate) that are absorbed and provide a significant metabolic fuel for intestinal enterocytes, and may provide protection against the development of colorectal cancer . Provision of a substrate for bacterial fermentation in the form of oligosaccharides, resistant starch, and non-starch polysaccharides alters the composition of the intestinal flora, enhancing the growth of beneficial bacteria at the expense of potential pathogens. Carbohydrates that occur in, or are added to, foods for this purpose are known as prebiotics. Foods that contain the bacteria (mainly Lactobacillus and Bifidobacterium spp.) themselves are known as probiotics. One of the advantages of breast-feeding over infant formula is that human milk is rich in prebiotic oligosaccharides that enhance the infant's ability to develop a desirable intestinal bacterial flora.

Carbohydrate Digestion and Absorption

The digestion of carbohydrates is by hydrolysis to liberate small oligosaccharides, then free mono- and disaccharides. The extent and speed with which a carbohydrate is hydrolyzed and the resultant monosaccharides absorbed is measured as the glycemic index; the increase in blood glucose after a test dose of the carbohydrate compared with that after an equivalent amount of glucose, either as a glucose solution or a reference source of carbohydrate such as white bread or boiled rice. Glucose and galactose have a glycemic index of 1, as do lactose, maltose, isomaltose, and trehalose, which give rise to these monosaccharides on hydrolysis. However, because plant cell walls are largely cellulose, which is not digested, intrinsic sugars in fruits and vegetables have a lower glycemic index. Other monosaccharides (e.g., fructose) and the sugar alcohols are absorbed less rapidly and have a lower glycemic index, as does sucrose, which yields glucose and fructose on hydrolysis.

The glycemic index of starch is variable and that of nonstarch polysaccharides is zero.

Carbohydrates with a high glycemic index lead to a greater secretion of insulin after a meal than do those with a lower glycemic index; this results in increased synthesis of fatty acids and triacylglycerol , and may therefore be a factor in the development of obesity and diabetes mellitus.

The enzymes that catalyze the hydrolysis of starch are amylases, which are secreted both in the saliva and the pancreatic juice. (Salivary amylase is sometimes known by its old name of ptyalin.) Both salivary and pancreatic amylases catalyze random hydrolysis of glycoside bonds, initially yielding dextrins and other oligosaccharides, then a mixture of glucose, maltose, and isomaltose (from the branch points in amylopectin).

The digestion of starch begins when food is chewed and continues for a time in the stomach. Hydrolysis of starch to sweet sugars in the mouth may be a factor in determining food and nutrient intake . The gastric juice is very acidic (about pH 1.5–2), and amylase is inactive at this pH; as the food bolus is mixed with gastric juice, starch digestion ceases. When the food leaves the stomach and enters the small intestine, it is neutralized by the alkaline pancreatic juice (pH 8.8) and bile (pH 8). Amylase secreted by the pancreas continues the digestion of starch begun by salivary amylase.

Starches can be classified as; (a) Rapidly hydrolyzed, with a glycemic index near 1; these are more or less completely hydrolyzed in the small intestine, (b)Slowly hydrolyzed, with a glycemic index significantly <1, so that a proportion remains in the gut lumen and is a substrate for bacterial fermentation in the colon, (c) Resistant to hydrolysis, with a glycemic index near to zero, so that most remains in the gut lumen and is a substrate for bacterial fermentation in the colon.

A proportion of the starch in foods is still enclosed by plant cell walls, which are mainly composed of cellulose. Cellulose is not digested by human enzymes, and therefore this starch is protected against digestion. Similarly, intrinsic sugars have a lower glycemic index than would be expected, because they are within intact cells. Uncooked starch is resistant to amylase action, because it is present as small insoluble granules. The process of cooking swells the starch granules, resulting in a gel on which amylase can act. However, as cooked starch cools, a proportion undergoes crystallization to a form that is again resistant to amylase action—this is part of the process of staling of starchy foods.

Like nonstarch polysaccharides, much of the resistant and slowly hydrolyzed starch is fermented by bacteria in the colon, and a proportion of the products of bacterial metabolism, including short-chain fatty acids, may be absorbed and metabolized. The enzymes that catalyze the hydrolysis of disaccharides (the disaccharidases) are located on the brush border of the intestinal mucosal cells; the resultant monosaccharides are absorbed together with dietary monosaccharides and glucose arising from the digestion of starch . There are four disaccharidases ; (a) Maltase, it catalyzes the hydrolysis of maltose to two molecules of glucose (b) Sucrase-isomaltase is a bifunctional enzyme that catalyzes the hydrolysis of sucrose to glucose and fructose, and of isomaltose to two molecules of glucose (c) Lactase, it catalyzes the hydrolysis of lactose to glucose and galactose and (d) Trehalase, it catalyzes the hydrolysis of trehalose to two molecules of glucose.

Deficiency of the enzyme lactase is common in the people of north European origin. In most other people, lactase is gradually lost through early adult life; alactasia. (In the absence of lactase, lactose cannot be absorbed, but remains in the intestinal lumen, where it is a substrate for bacterial fermentation to lactate . This results in a considerable increase in the osmolality of the intestinal contents, since 1 mol of lactose yields 4 mol of lactate and 4 mol of protons. In addition, bacterial fermentation produces carbon dioxide, methane, and hydrogen, and the result of consuming a moderate amount of lactose is an explosive watery diarrhea with severe abdominal pain. Even the relatively small amounts of lactose in milk may upset people with a complete deficiency of lactase. Such people can normally tolerate yogurt and other fermented milk products, since much of the lactose has been converted to lactic acid. Fortunately, for people who suffer from alactasia, milk is the only significant source of lactose in the diet, so it is relatively easy to avoid consuming it. Lactose is widely used in manufacture of pharmaceuticals, but the small amounts consumed seem to be tolerated by people who are alactasic.

Rarely, people may lack sucrase-isomaltase, maltase, or trehalase. This may either be a genetic lack of the enzyme, or an acquired loss as a result of intestinal infection, when all four disaccharidases are lost. These people are intolerant of the sugar(s) that cannot be hydrolyzed and suffer in the same way as alactasic subjects given lactose. It is relatively easy to avoid maltose and trehalose, since there are few sources in the diet. People who lack sucrase have a more serious problem, since as well as the obvious sugar in cakes, biscuits, and jams, many manufactured foods contain added sucrose.

Genetic lack of sucrase-isomaltase is very common among the Inuit of North America. This caused no problems on their traditional diet, since they had no significant sources of sucrose or isomaltose. With the adoption of a more Western diet, sucrose-induced diarrhea has become a significant cause of undernutrition among infants and children.

There are two separate mechanisms for the absorption of monosaccharides in the small intestine .Glucose and galactose are absorbed by a sodium-dependent active process. The sodium pump and the sodium/potassium ATPase as well as sodium secreted in the alkaline pancreatic juice, create a sodium gradient across the membrane. The sodium ions then enter the cell together with glucose or galactose. These two monosaccharides are carried by the same transport protein and compete with each other for intestinal absorption.

Other monosaccharides are absorbed by carrier-mediated diffusion; there are at least three distinct carrier proteins, one for fructose, one for other monosaccharides, and one for sugar alcohols. Because they are not actively transported, fructose and sugar alcohols are only absorbed to a limited extent, and after a moderately high intake, a significant amount will avoid absorption, and remain in the intestinal lumen, acting as a substrate for colon bacteria and, like unabsorbed disaccharides in people with disaccharidase deficiency, causing abdominal pain and diarrhea.

Digestion and Absorption of Fats

The major fats in the diet are triacylglycerols and, to a lesser extent, phospholipids. Lipids are hydrophobic and have to be emulsified to very small droplets (micelles) before they can be absorbed. This emulsification is achieved by hydrolysis of triacylglycerols to mono- and diacylglycerols and free fatty acids, and also by the action of the bile salts.

Dietary lipids are classified in four groups of metabolically important compounds;

(a) Triacylglycerols (sometimes also known as triglycerides), in which glycerol is esterified to three fatty acids . These are the oils and fats of the diet, which provide between 30% and 45% of average energy intake. The difference between oils and fats is that oils are liquid at room temperature, whereas fats are solid.

(b) Phospholipids, in which glycerol is esterified to two fatty acids, with a hydrophilic group esterified to carbon-3 by a phosphate diester bond . Phospho- lipids are major constituents of cell membranes.

(c) Steroids, including cholesterol, a variety of plant sterols and stanols and extremely small amounts of steroid hormones . Chemically, these are completely different from triacylglycerols and phospholipids.

(d) A variety of other compounds, including vitamin A and carotenes, vitamin D, vitamin E, and vitamin K. They are absorbed in lipid micelles, and their absorption depends on an adequate intake of fat.

There are a number of different fatty acids, differing in both the length of the carbon chain and whether or not they have one or more double bonds (–CH=CH–) in the chain . Those with no double bonds are saturated fatty acids; the carbon chain is completely saturated with hydrogen. Those with double bonds are unsaturated fatty acids; the carbon chain is not completely saturated with hydrogen. Fatty acids with one double bond are known as monounsaturated, while those with two or more double bonds are known as polyunsaturated.

While it is the fatty acids that are saturated or unsaturated, it is common to discuss saturated and unsaturated fats. Although not really correct, it is a useful shorthand, reflecting the fact that fats from different sources contain a greater or lesser proportion of saturated and unsaturated fatty acids.

Many fatty acids have trivial names, often derived from the source from which they were originally isolated; thus oleic acid was first isolated from olive oil, stearic acid from beef tallow, palmitic acid from palm oil, linoleic and linolenic acids from linseed oil. All have systematic chemical names based on the number of carbon atoms in the chain and the number and position of double bonds.

In the nutritionally important unsaturated fatty acids, the carbon–carbon double bonds are in the cis configuration. The trans isomers of unsaturated fatty acids occur in foods to some extent, both as a result of hydrogenation of unsaturated oils to more solid fats for food manufacture and also naturally occurring in fat from ruminants, as a result of rumen bacterial fermentation. They do not have the desirable biological actions of the cis isomers, and indeed there is evidence that trans fatty acids have adverse effects. It is recommended that trans unsaturated fatty acids should not exceed 1% of energy intake.

Table: Fatty Acid Nomenclature

Double Bonds

	C Atoms	Number	First	Shorthand
Saturated				
Butyric	4	0	–	C4:0
Caproic	6	0	–	C6:0
Caprylic	8	0	–	C8:0
Capric	10	0	–	C10:0
Lauric	12	0	–	C12:0
Myristic	14	0	–	C14:0
Palmitic	16	0	–	C16:0
Stearic	18	0	–	C18:0

	C Atoms	Number	First	Shorthand
Arachidic	20	0	–	C20:0
Behenic	22	0	–	C22:0
Lignoceric	24	0	–	C24:0
Monounsaturated				
Palmitoleic	16	1	7	C16:1 ω7
Oleic	18	1	9	C18:1 ω9
Cetoleic	22	1	11	C22:1 ω11
Nervonic	24	1	9	C24:1 ω9
Polyunsaturated				
Linoleic	18	2	6	C18:2 ω6
α-Linolenic	18	3	3	C18:3 ω3
γ-Linolenic	18	3	6	C18:3 ω6
Arachidonic	20	4	6	C20:4 ω6
Eicosapentaenoic	20	5	3	C20:5 ω3
Docosatetraenoic	22	4	6	C22:4 ω6
Docosapentaenoic	22	5	3	C22:5 ω3
Docosapentaenoic	22	5	6	C22:5 ω6
Docosahexaenoic	22	6	3	C22:6 ω3

Polyunsaturated fatty acids have two main functions in the body:

Maintaining membrane fluidity as major constituents of the phospholipids in cell membranes.

Function as local hormones (paracrine agents) as precursors for the synthesis of a group of compounds known as eicosanoids, including prostaglandins, prostacyclins, and thromboxanes, being secreted into the extracellular fluid and acting on nearby cells.

The polyunsaturated fatty acids can be interconverted to a limited extent in the body, but there is a requirement for a dietary intake of linoleic acid (C18:2 ω6) and linolenic acid (C18:3 ω3), since these two, which can each be considered to be the precursor of a family of related fatty acids and eicosanoids, cannot be synthesized in the body.

An intake of polyunsaturated fatty acids greater than needed to meet physiological requirements may confer benefits in terms of lowering the plasma concentration of cholesterol and reducing the risk of atherosclerosis and ischemic heart disease. The requirement is less than 1% of energy intake, but it is recommended that 6% of energy intake should come from polyunsaturated fatty acids .

High intakes of the long-chain ω3 polyunsaturated fatty acids (as found in fish oils) may additionally provide protection against thrombosis, since they form the ω3-series eicosanoids, which inhibit platelet cohesiveness. However, the same enzymes are involved in the metabolism of both ω3 and ω6 polyunsaturated fatty acids to form eicosanoids, and the two families of fatty acids compete with each other for metabolism. This means that the balance between ω3 and ω6 polyunsaturated fatty acids in the diet is important; excessive intakes of one group will lead to reduced formation of the other group of eicosanoids.

Phospholipids are lipids that contain a phosphate group, they consist of glycerol esterified to two fatty acids, one of which (esterified to carbon-2 of glycerol) is polyunsaturated. The third hydroxyl group of glycerol is esterified to phosphate, which in turn is esterified to one of a variety of compounds, including the amino acid serine, ethanolamine (which is formed from serine), choline (which is formed from ethanolamine), and inositol. A phospholipid lacking the group esterified to the phosphate is known as a phosphatidic acid, and the complete phospholipids are called phosphatidyl serine, phosphatidyl ethanolamine, phosphatidyl choline (also called lecithin), phosphatidyl inositol, etc.

Phospholipids in cell membranes form a lipid bilayer, with the hydrophobic fatty acid chains inside, and the hydrophilic groups outside. Various proteins may be embedded in the membrane at one surface or the other, or may span the membrane (transmembrane proteins) as either transport proteins or receptors for hormones and neurotransmitters . The polyunsaturated fatty acids esterified at carbon-2 of glycerol in phospholipids are essential for membrane fluidity; neither saturated fatty acids nor the trans isomers of polyunsaturated fatty acids will pack to form an adequately fluid membrane. Other lipids, including cholesterol and vitamin E are dissolved in the hydrophobic interior of the membrane and are essential to its function.

In addition to its structural role, phosphatidyl inositol has a specialized function in membranes, acting as the source of inositol trisphosphate and diacylglycerol that are produced as intracellular second messengers in response to fast-acting hormones and neurotransmitters.

Cholesterol and the Steroids

Steroids are chemically completely different from triacylglycerols or phospholipids . The parent compound of all the steroids in the body is cholesterol; different steroids are then formed by replacing one or more of the hydrogens with hydroxyl groups or oxo-groups, and in some cases by modifying the side chain.

Apart from cholesterol, which is important in membrane structure and the synthesis of bile salts steroids are slow-acting hormones. Vitamin D is a derivative of cholesterol, and can also be considered to be a steroid hormone. The cholesterol that is required for membrane synthesis, and the very much smaller amount required for the synthesis of steroid hormones, may either be synthesized in the body or provided by the diet; average intakes are of the order of 200–500 mg/day.

An elevated plasma concentration of cholesterol (in low density lipoproteins); is a risk factor for atherosclerosis and ischemic heart disease. The dietary intake of total and saturated fat , the intake of compounds such as sitosterol and cholestanol that inhibit the absorption of dietary cholesterol and the reabsorption of cholesterol secreted in bile, or the reabsorption of bile salts themselves .

Digestion and Absorption of Triacylglycerols

The digestion of triacylglycerols begins with lipase secreted by the tongue; lingual lipase may be important in permitting the detection of fat in the diet, and hence in determining food choices . However, it makes only a marginal contribution to overall triacylglycerol hydrolysis, which continues in the stomach, where gastric lipase is secreted. Hydrolysis of the fatty acids esterified to carbons 1 and 3 of the triacylglycerol results in the liberation of free fatty acids and 2-mono-acylglycerol . These have both hydrophobic and hydrophilic regions, and will therefore emulsify the lipid into increasingly small droplets. Triacylglycerol hydrolysis continues in the small intestine, catalyzed by pancreatic lipase, which requires a further pancreatic protein, colipase, for activity. Monoacylglycerols are hydrolyzed to glycerol and free fatty acids by pancreatic esterase in the intestinal lumen and intracellular lipase within intestinal mucosal cells.

The final emulsification of dietary lipids into micelles (droplets that are small enough to be absorbed across the intestinal mucosa) is achieved by the action of the bile salts. They are synthesized from cholesterol in the liver, and secreted, together with phospholipids and cholesterol, by the gall bladder. Some 2 g of cholesterol and 30 g of bile salts are secreted by the gall bladder each day, almost all of which is reabsorbed, so that the total fecal output of steroids and bile salts is 0.2–1 g/day.

The primary bile salts (those synthesized in the liver) are conjugates of chenodeoxycholic acid and cholic acid with taurine or glycine . Intestinal bacteria catalyze deconjugation and further metabolism to yield the secondary bile salts, lithocholic and deoxycholic acids. These are also absorbed from the gut, and are reconjugated in the liver and secreted in the bile.

The bile salts can be bound physically by insoluble nonstarch polysaccharide in the intestinal lumen, so that they cannot be reabsorbed. This is the basis of the cholesterol-lowering effect of moderately high intakes of nonstarch polysaccharide if the bile salts are not reabsorbed and reutilized, then there must be further synthesis from cholesterol in the liver, thus depleting body cholesterol.

Under normal conditions, the concentration of cholesterol in bile, relative to that of bile salts and phospholipids, is such that cholesterol is at or near its limit of solubility. It only requires a relatively small increase in the concentration of cholesterol in bile for it to crystallize out, resulting in the formation of gallstones. Obesity and high-fat diets (especially diets high in saturated fat, which increase the synthesis of cholesterol in the liver) are associated with a considerably increased incidence of gallstones.

The finely emulsified lipid micelles, containing free fatty acids, monoacylglycerol, phospholipids, cholesterol, and fat-soluble vitamins, together with a small amount of intact triacylglycerol, are absorbed across the intestinal wall into the mucosal cells. There are membrane transport proteins for fatty acids and cholesterol.

Inside the enterocyte, fatty acids are reesterified to form triacylglycerol , and cholesterol is esterified. Newly esterified triacylglycerol, cholesterol esters, and lipid-soluble vitamins are packaged with proteins synthesized in the enterocyte to form chylomicrons, which are secreted into the lacteal in the center of the villus, and enter the lymphatic system, which drains into the bloodstream at the thoracic duct. In response to the action of insulin, lipoprotein lipase at the surface of blood vessel endothelial cells in adipose tissue and muscle is activated and catalyzes the hydrolysis of chylomicron triacylglycerol. The resultant fatty acids are taken up by adipose tissue and reesterified for storage; in muscle the fatty acids may either be used as a metabolic fuel or be reesterified for storage between muscle fibers. A proportion of the fatty acid released by lipoprotein lipase remains in the bloodstream and is taken up by the liver, where it is reesterified and incorporated into very low density lipoprotein.

The triacylglycerol-depleted chylomicron remnants are taken up by the liver through receptor-mediated endocytosis, and most of the residual lipid is secreted in very low- density lipoprotein, together with triacylglycerol synthesized in the liver.

Digestion and Absorption of Proteins

Proteins are polypeptides; polymers of amino acids linked by peptide bonds. Unlike starch and glycogen, which are polymers of only a single type of monomer unit (glucose), proteins contain 21 different amino acids that are incorporated during synthesis (Section 9.2) as well as a number of others that are formed as a result of postsynthetic modification. Since any

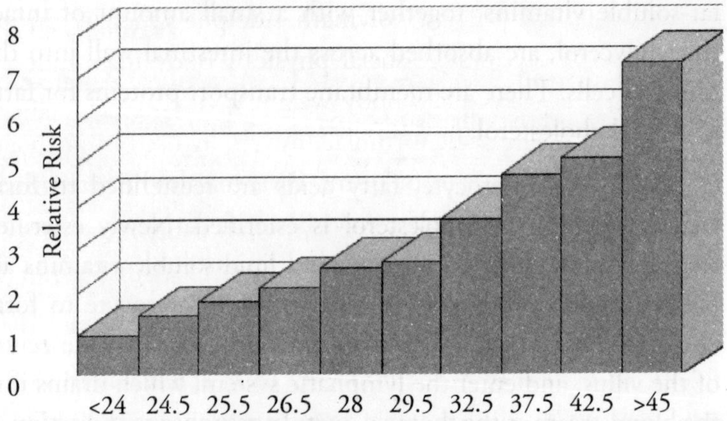

Fig.: The incidence of gallstones with obesity (body mass index = weight [kg]/height [m^2]; the desirable range is 20–25

individual polypeptide chain may contain 50–1000 amino acids, there is an almost infinite possible variety of proteins. There are some 30,000–40,000 different proteins and polypeptides in the human body; each has a specific sequence of amino acids.

Small proteins have a molecular mass of about $50–100 \times 10^3$, while some of the large complex proteins have a molecular mass of up to 10^4 or more. Smaller polypeptides (containing between 3 and 50 amino acids) are important in the regulation of metabolism.

The Body Mass Index

The body mass index (BMI), or Quetelet index, is a statistical measurement which compares a person's weight and height. Though it does not actually measure the percentage of body fat, it is used to estimate a healthy body weight based on how tall a person is. Due to its ease of measurement and calculation, it is the most widely used diagnostic tool to identify weight problems within a population, usually whether individuals are underweight, overweight or obese. It was invented between 1830 and 1850 by the Belgian polymath Adolphe Quetelet during the course of developing "social physics". Body mass index is defined as the individual's body weight divided by the square of his or her height. The formulae universally used in medicine produce a unit of measure of kg/m^2. BMI can also be determined using a BMI chart, which displays BMI as a function of weight (horizontal axis) and height (vertical axis) using contour lines for different values of BMI or colours for different BMI categories.

$$\text{SI Units} \quad BMI = \frac{mass(kg)}{height^2(m^2)}$$

A graph of body mass index is shown below. The dashed lines represent subdivisions within a major class. For instance the "Underweight" classification is further divided into "severe," "moderate," and "mild" subclasses. Based on WHO data.

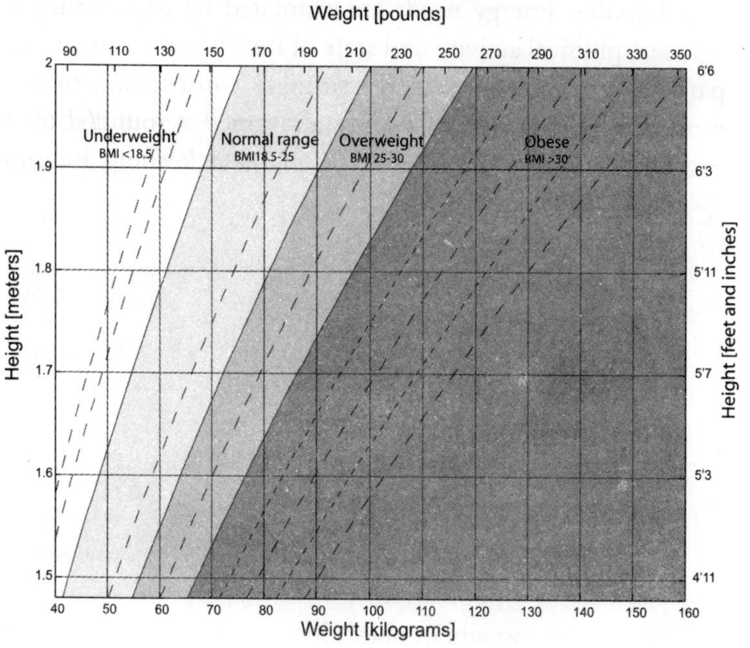

Determine your BMI using the formula.

$$BMI = \frac{mass(kg)}{height^2(m^2)}$$

Subject: Male 5'8", Actual Weight = 56kg

Note: 1 inch = 2.54 cms; 1m = 100cms; 1 kg = 2.2 pounds

5 × 12 = 60 inches + 8 = 68 inches × 2.54 = 172.72 cm/100 = 1.7272 multiply by itself = 2.98.

BMI = 56kg/2.98 = <u>18.79 (Normal based on the table ahead)</u>

These ranges of BMI values are valid only as statistical categories when applied to adults, and do not predict health.

Voluntary (muscular) and involuntary (metabolic processes) activities of the body require energy. Energy comes from the oxidation of foods and is measured in terms of calories or kilojoules. Energy needs are estimated by considering the age, sex, physical activity and state of health such as pregnancy, pathologic conditions, etc. To simplify construction of daily food plan, the estimated energy allowance is rounded-off to nearest 50 kcal. Diet Should be planned keeping in mind specific need of subjects.

Category	BMI Range: kg/m^2	BMI Prime	Mass (Weight) of a 1.8 Metres (5 ft. 11 in.) Person with this BMI
Severely underweight	less than 16.5	less than 0.66	under 53.5 kilograms (8.42 st; 118 lb)
Underweight	from 16.5 to 18.4	from 0.66 to 0.73	between 53.5 and 60 kilograms (8.42 and 9.45 st; 118 and 132 lb)
Normal	from 18.5 to 24.9	from 0.74 to 0.99	between 60 and 81 kilograms (9.4 and 13 st; 130 and 180 lb)
Overweight	from 25 to 30	from 1.0 to 1.2	between 81 and 97 kilograms (12.8 and 15.3 st; 180 and 210 lb)
Obese Class I	from 30.1 to 34.9	from 1.21 to 1.4	between 97 and 113 kilograms (15.3 and 17.8 st; 210 and 250 lb)
Obese Class II	from 35 to 40	from 1.41 to 1.6	between 113 and 130 kilograms (17.8 and 20.5 st; 250 and 290 lb)
Obese Class III	over 40	over 1.6	over 130 kilograms (20 st; 290 lb)

The Amino Acids

Chemically, all the amino acids all have the same basic structure; an amino group (–NH_3^+) and a carboxylic acid group (–COO^-) attached to the same carbon atom (the α-carbon); what differs between the amino acids is the nature of the other group that is attached to the α-carbon. In the simplest amino acid, glycine, there are two hydrogen atoms, while in all other amino acids there is one hydrogen atom and a side chain, varying in chemical complexity from the simple methyl group (–CH_3) of alanine to the aromatic ring structures of phenylalanine, tyrosine, and tryptophan. The twenty-first amino acid is selenocysteine, the selenium analogue of cysteine.

Nine of the amino acids are dietary essentials that cannot be synthesized in the body ; The amino acids can be classified according to the chemical nature of the side chain: whether it is hydrophobic or hydrophilic and the nature of thc group:

Small hydrophobic amino acids: glycine, alanine, proline

Large hydrophobic, branched-chain amino acids: leucine, isoleucine, valine

Aromatic amino acids: phenylalanine, tyrosine, tryptophan

Sulfur-containing amino acids: cysteine and methionine

Neutral hydrophilic amino acids: serine and threonine

Acidic amino acids: glutamic and aspartic acids (the salts of these acids are glutamate and aspartate, respectively)

Amides of the acidic amino acids: glutamine and asparagine

Basic amino acids: lysine, arginine, histidine

In addition to the three-letter abbreviations that are commonly used for the amino acids, there is a single-letter code for each that is generally used for showing protein sequences.

Proteins are composed of linear chains of amino acids, joined by condensation of the carboxyl group of one with the amino group of another, to form a peptide bond. The sequence of amino acids in a protein is its primary structure. It is different for each protein, although proteins that are closely related to each other often have very similar primary structures. The primary structure of a protein is determined by the gene containing the information for that protein. Polypeptide chains fold up in a variety of ways, stabilized by hydrogen bonds between the oxygen of one peptide bond and the nitrogen of another. Interactions between the side chains of the amino acids determine which of the following patterns of secondary structure any given region of a protein adopts:

α-Helix, in which the peptide backbone of the protein adopts a spiral (helix) form, the hydrogen bonds are formed between peptide bonds that are near each other in the primary sequence, β-Pleated sheet, in which regions of the polypeptide chain lie alongside one another, forming a "corrugated" or pleated surface. The hydrogen bonds are between peptide bonds in different parts of the primary sequence, and the regions of polypeptide chain forming a pleated sheet may run parallel or antiparallel, Hairpins and loops, in which small regions of the polypeptide chain form very tight bends, Random coil, in which there is no recognizable organized structure. Although this appears to be random, for any one protein the shape of a random coil region will always be the same. A protein may have several regions of α-helix, β-pleated sheet (with the peptide chains running parallel or antiparallel), hairpins, and random coil, all in the same molecule.

Having formed regions of secondary structure, the whole protein molecule then folds up into a compact shape. This is the third (tertiary) level of structure and is largely the result of interactions of the side chains of the amino acids with each other and their environment. Proteins in an aqueous medium in the cell generally adopt a tertiary structure in which hydrophobic side chains are inside the molecule and can interact with each other, while hydrophilic side chains are exposed to interact with water. In contrast, proteins that are embedded in membranes have a hydrophobic region on the outside to interact with the membrane lipids.

Two further interactions between amino acid side chains may be involved in the tertiary structure, in this case forming covalent bonds between regions of the peptide chain;

(a) The ε-amino group on the side chain of lysine can form a peptide bond with the carboxyl group on the side chain of aspartate or glutamate. This is nutritionally important, since the side chain peptide bond is not hydrolyzed by digestive enzymes, and the lysine, which is an essential amino acid, is not available for absorption.

(b) The sulfydryl (–SH) groups of two cysteine molecules may be oxidized to form a disulfide bridge between two parts of the protein chain.

Some proteins consist of more than one polypeptide chain; the way in which the chains interact with each other, after each has formed its secondary and tertiary structures, is the quaternary structure of the protein. Interactions between the subunits of multi-subunit proteins, involving changes in quaternary structure and the conformation of the protein, are important in a number of regulatory enzymes.

Because of their compact secondary and tertiary structures, most proteins are resistant to digestive enzymes, few bonds are accessible to the proteolytic enzymes that catalyze hydrolysis of peptide bonds. However, apart from covalent links formed by reaction between the side chains of lysine and aspartate or glutamate, and disulfide bridges, the native structure of proteins is maintained by relatively weak noncovalent forces: ionic interactions, hydrogen bonding, and van der Waals forces.

Denaturation of a protein is the loss of its compact secondary and tertiary structures, opening out the molecule so that it becomes insoluble (and in the case of an enzyme, loses its catalytic activity). Denatured proteins are susceptible to the action of digestive enzymes, so that denaturation is an important precursor to protein digestion. The relatively weak bonds that maintain the native structure of proteins can be disrupted by heat and extremes of pH, so that both cooking and gastric acid are important in protein digestion.

Protein Digestion

Protein digestion occurs by hydrolysis of the peptide bonds between amino acids. There are two main classes of protein digestive enzymes (proteases) with different specificities for the amino acids forming the peptide bond to be hydrolyzed;

(a) Endopeptidases cleave proteins by hydrolyzing peptide bonds between specific amino acids throughout the molecule.

(b) Exopeptidases remove amino acids one at a time from either the amino or carboxyl end of the molecule, again by the hydrolysis of the peptide bond.

Table 4.2 Protein Digestive Enzymes

	Secreted by	Specificity
Endopeptidases Pepsin	Gastric mucosa	Adjacent to aromatic amino acid, leucine, or methionine
Trypsin	Pancreas	Lysine or arginine esters
Chymotrypsin	Pancreas	Aromatic esters
Elastase	Pancreas	Neutral eliphatic esters
Enteropeptidase	Intestinal mucosa	Trypsinogen→trypsin
Exopeptidases		
Carboxypeptidases	Pancreas Intestinal mucosa	Carboxy-terminal amino acids
Aminopeptidases	Mucosal brush border	Amino-terminal amino acids
Tripeptidases	Mucosal brush border	Tripeptides
Dipeptidases		Dipeptides

The first enzymes to act on dietary proteins are the endopeptidases: pepsin in the gastric juice and trypsin, chymotrypsin, and elastase in the small intestine. The result of the combined action of the endopeptidases is that the large protein molecules are broken down into smaller polypeptides with a large number of amino and carboxyl terminals for the exopeptidases to act on. There are two classes of exopeptidase; Carboxypeptidases, secreted in the pancreatic juice, release amino acids from the free carboxyl terminal of peptides and Aminopeptidases, secreted by the intestinal mucosal cells, release amino acids from the amino terminal of peptides. Both amino- and carboxypeptidases continue to act until the final product is a di- or tripeptide, which is hydrolyzed by di- and tripeptidases inside the mucosal cell. The proteases are secreted as inactive precursors (zymogens); this is essential if they are not to digest themselves and tissue proteins before they are secreted. In each case, the active site of the enzyme is masked by a small region of the peptide chain that has to be removed for the enzyme to have activity. This is achieved by hydrolysis of a specific peptide bond in the precursor molecule, releasing the blocking peptide and revealing the active site of the enzyme.

Pepsin is secreted in the gastric juice as pepsinogen, which is activated by the action of gastric acid, and also by the action of already activated pepsin. In the small intestine, trypsinogen, the precursor of trypsin, is activated by the action of a specific enzyme, enteropeptidase (enterokinase), which is secreted by the duodenal epithelial cells; trypsin can then activate chymotrypsinogen to chymotrypsin, proelastase to elastase, procarboxypeptidase to carboxypeptidase, and proaminopeptidase to aminopeptidase.

Absorption of the Products of Protein Digestion

The end product of the action of endopeptidases and exopeptidases is a mixture of free amino acids, di- and tripeptides, and oligopeptides.

Free amino acids are absorbed across the intestinal mucosa by sodium-dependent active transport, as occurs in the absorption of glucose and galactose . There are a number of different amino acid transport systems, with specificity for the chemical nature of the side chain (large or small neutral, acidic, or basic). Similar group-specific amino acid transporters occur in the renal tubules (for reabsorption of amino acids filtered at the glomerulus) and for uptake of amino acids into tissues. The various amino acids carried by any one transporter compete with each other for absorption and tissue uptake.

Dipeptides and tripeptides enter the brush border of the intestinal mucosal cells, where they are hydrolyzed to free amino acids, which are then transported into the blood- stream. Patients with genetic defects of one or other of the amino acid transporters can still absorb dipeptides and so have a limited dietary source of all the amino acids.

Relatively large peptides can be absorbed intact, either by uptake into mucosal epithelial cells (the transcellular route) or by passing between epithelial cells (the paracellular route). These peptides may be large enough to stimulate antibody production; this is the basis of allergic reactions to foods. In infants, there is greater absorption of intact small proteins and oligopeptides than in adults; this permits the infant to gain passive immunity by absorbing immunoglobulins in breast milk. However, it also means that early exposure to foreign proteins can result in the development of food allergy; cow's milk, egg, and peanut proteins are common food allergens.

The Absorption of Vitamins and Minerals

In addition to compounds that enter the small intestine from the diet, a number of vitamins and other compounds are secreted in the bile, then reabsorbed from the small intestine; a process of enterohepatic circulation. For example, the total amount of cholesterol entering the gut is some four-to fivefold higher than the dietary intake, so that inhibition of cholesterol absorption has a considerably greater effect than might be expected . Folate and vitamin B12 undergo similar enterohepatic circulation. In the case of vitamin B12, this serves to remove degradation products and metabolites that have antivitamin activity, since the intestinal binding protein that is required for vitamin B12 absorption (intrinsic factor) binds only biologically active vitamin B12 and none of its analogs.

Absorption of Fat-soluble Vitamins and Cholesterol

Absorption of the fat-soluble vitamins (A, D, E, and K) depends on an adequate total amount of fat in the diet, because they are absorbed dissolved in the core of lipid micelles and then incorporated into chylomicrons together with reesterified fatty acids . Vitamins D and E and carotenes are absorbed passively by diffusion. Vitamin A enters enterocytes by carrier-mediated transport followed by esterification to permit accumulation; when the carrier is saturated, there is also passive uptake of the vitamin. Vitamin K is transported into enterocytes by an ATP-dependent transporter.

Cholesterol enters enterocytes by carrier-mediated transport. Plant sterols and stanols compete with cholesterol for the transport protein, thus reducing the absorption of both dietary cholesterol and that secreted in the bile. They also inhibit the esterification of cholesterol; any unesterified cholesterol in the enterocyte, as well as unesterified plant sterols and stanols, is actively transported out of the enterocyte back into the intestinal lumen by an ATP-binding transport protein.

Absorption of Water-soluble Vitamins

The absorption of water-soluble vitamins requires a transport protein at the luminal surface of the mucosal cell; this may involve active or passive transport, and may be followed by metabolic trapping to permit accumulation. In some cases, active transport is involved in the efflux of the vitamin from the enterocyte into the bloodstream.

Thiamin (vitamin B1) enters the enterocyte by active transport via a proton-pumping ATPase. Some is phosphorylated intracellularly, and there is Na^+-dependent active transport into the bloodstream. The active transport of thiamin out of the enterocyte into the bloodstream is inhibited by alcohol, which, together with a poor diet, explains the relatively common occurrence of thiamin deficiency in alcoholics.

Riboflavin (vitamin B2) enters the enterocyte by Na^+-dependent active transport, followed by metabolic trapping as riboflavin monophosphate.

The niacin vitamers, nicotinic acid and nicotinamide enter the enterocyte by Na^+-dependent active transport.

Vitamin B6 enters the enterocyte by carrier-mediated passive transport, followed by metabolic trapping as pyridoxal phosphate. However, much is dephosphorylated by alkaline phosphatase at the serosal surface of the cell, so that it is mainly pyridoxal rather than pyridoxal phosphate that enters the bloodstream.

Dietary folate is a mixture of derivatives with different lengths of a poly-γ-glutamyl side chain. In the intestinal lumen, the side chain is removed by conjugase (a zinc-dependent enzyme), and folate monoglutamate enters the enterocyte by carrier-mediated passive uptake, followed by reduction and methylation, so that what enters the bloodstream is mainly methyl-tetrahydrofolate.

Despite their very different structures, biotin and pantothenic acid enter the enterocyte using the same Na^+-dependent active transport protein.

Vitamin C enters the enterocyte by Na^+-dependent active transport. This transport protein is found elsewhere in the gastrointestinal tract, and a modest amount of vitamin C can be absorbed in the mouth.

Very small amounts of vitamin B12 can be absorbed by passive diffusion across the intestinal mucosa, but under normal conditions this is insignificant, accounting for less than 1% of a large oral dose; the major route of vitamin B12 absorption is by way of attachment to a specific binding protein in the intestinal lumen. This binding protein is "intrinsic factor," so called because in the early studies of pernicious anemia, it has been found that two curative factors were involved; an extrinsic or dietary factor, which we now know to be vitamin B12, and an intrinsic or endogenously produced factor. Intrinsic factor is a small glycoprotein secreted by the parietal cells of the gastric mucosa, which also secrete hydrochloric acid.

Both gastric acid and pepsin have a role in vitamin B12 absorption, serving to release the vitamin from the proteins it is bound to in foods. Atrophic gastritis is a relatively common problem of advancing age; in the early stages there is impaired acid secretion but more or less normal secretion of intrinsic factor. This can result in vitamin B12 depletion due to failure to release the vitamin from dietary proteins, but the absorption of free vitamin B12 is unaffected. Inhibition of gastric acid secretion to treat gastric ulcers and hiatus hernia will also impair the release of vitamin B12 from dietary proteins, but there is no evidence that even prolonged use of the proton pump inhibiting drugs results in vitamin B12 deficiency.

In the stomach, vitamin B12 binds to cobalophilin, a binding protein secreted in the saliva. Cobalophilin is hydrolyzed in the duodenum, releasing the vitamin B12 for binding to intrinsic factor. Pancreatic insufficiency can therefore be a factor in the development of vitamin B12 deficiency, since failure to hydrolyze cobalophilin will result in the excretion of cobalophilin-bound vitamin B12 rather than transfer to intrinsic factor. Intrinsic factor binds biologically active vitamin B12, but not analogs that have no biological activity. Considerably more intrinsic factor is normally secreted than is needed for the binding and absorption of dietary vitamin B12, which requires only about 1% of the total intrinsic factor available.

Vitamin B12 is absorbed from the distal third of the ileum by receptor-mediated endocytosis. There are intrinsic factor–vitamin B12 binding sites on the brush border of the mucosal cells in this region; free intrinsic factor does not interact with these receptors. The absorption of vitamin B12 is limited by the number of binding sites in the ileal mucosa, so that not more than about 1–1.5 μg of a single oral dose of the vitamin is absorbed.

Within the mucosal cell, the vitamin is released by lysosomal proteolysis of intrinsic factor, and is bound to transcobalamin II, a binding protein synthesized in the enterocytes, and stored in vesicles destined for export from the cell. In plasma, vitamin B12 circulates bound to transcobalamin I, which is required for tissue uptake of the vitamin, and transcobalamin II, which seems to be a storage form of the vitamin.

There is a considerable enterohepatic circulation of vitamin B12. Vitamin B12 and its biologically inactive metabolites are transferred from peripheral tissues to the liver bound to transcobalamin III. They are then secreted into the bile, bound to cobalophilins; 3–8 μg of vitamin B12 may be secreted in the bile each day, about the same as the average dietary intake. Like dietary vitamin B12 bound to salivary cobalophilin, the biliary cobalophilins are hydrolyzed in the duodenum, and the vitamin binds to intrinsic factor, thereby permitting reabsorption in the ileum. While cobalophilins and transcorrin III have low specificity, and will bind a variety of vitamin B12 analogs, intrinsic factor binds only cobalamins, and thus only the biologically active vitamin will be reabsorbed to any significant extent.

Absorption of Minerals

Mineral ions require a transport protein at the luminal surface of the mucosal cell and are accumulated inside the mucosal cell by binding to intracellular proteins. Transfer from mucosal cells into the bloodstream is usually by ATP-dependent active transport, commonly onto a plasma-binding protein. Genetic defects of the intracellular binding proteins or the active transport systems at the basal membrane of the mucosal cell can result in deficiency despite an apparently adequate intake of the mineral . The absorption of calcium is dependent on vitamin D . Synthesis of calbindin, the intracellular binding protein that is required for accumulation of calcium, requires the nuclear action of vitamin D, so that when vitamin D-deficient animals are repleted with the vitamin there is a significant time lag before calcium absorption increases.

The calcium transport protein only migrates from intracellular vesicles to the cell surface, to permit uptake of calcium, in response to rapid (cell-surface receptor-mediated) actions of vitamin D.

The absorption of many minerals is affected by other compounds present in the intestinal lumen. Reducing compounds can enhance the absorption of iron and chelating compounds enhance the absorption of other minerals. For example, zinc absorption is dependent on the secretion by the pancreas of a zinc-binding ligand (tryptophan metabolite picolinic acid). Failure to synthesize and secrete this zinc-binding ligand as a result of a genetic disease leads to the condition of acrodermatitis enteropathica; functional zinc deficiency despite an apparently adequate intake.

Diets based on unleavened wheat bread contain a relatively large amount of phytic acid (inositol hexaphosphate), which can bind calcium, iron, and zinc to form insoluble complexes that are not absorbed. Phytases in yeast catalyze dephosphorylation of phytate to products that do not chelate the minerals. Polyphenols, especially tannic acid in tea, can also chelate iron and other minerals, reducing their absorption, and large amounts of free fatty acids in the gut lumen can impair the absorption of calcium and magnesium, by forming insoluble soaps.

So far about 10%–15% of total dietary iron is absorbed, depending on the state of body iron reserves, and as little as 1%–5% of the inorganic iron in plant foods. Heme iron in meat is better absorbed by a separate transport system .

Inorganic iron is absorbed only in the Fe^{2+} (reduced) form. This means that a variety of reducing agents present in the intestinal lumen together with dietary iron will enhance its absorption. The most effective of such compounds is vitamin C, while intakes of 40–100 mg/day of vitamin C are more than adequate to meet requirements, an intake of 25–50 mg/meal is sometimes recommended to enhance iron absorption.

Alcohol, fructose, and a number of organic acids also enhance iron absorption.

Inorganic iron enters the mucosal cells by a proton-linked active transport mechanism, while there is a separate transporter for the uptake of heme. Heme iron is released as Fe^{2+} by the action of heme oxygenase. Iron can only leave the mucosal cell via the transport protein ferroportin, and only if there is free apotransferrin in the bloodstream to oxidize it to Fe^{3+} and bind it. The activity of ferroportin (and possibly also that of the divalent metal transporter) is downregulated by hepcidin, a peptide secreted by the liver. In response to anemia, hypoxia, or hemorrhage, hepcidin secretion is reduced and the activity of ferroportin increases, so that more iron can enter the bloodstream from the mucosal cells. Iron in the mucosal cell that is not transported out by ferroportin is oxidized to Fe^{3+} and bound to ferritin. It is then lost into the intestinal lumen when the cells are shed at the tip of the villus.

This mucosal barrier to the absorption of iron has a protective function. There is no pathway for excretion of iron from the body, although there are obligatory losses in shed skin and intestinal cells; thus iron reserves are controlled by regulation of intestinal absorption. About 10% of the population are genetically susceptible to iron overload (hemochromatosis). This is a serious condition, with deposition of inappropriately large amounts of iron in hemosiderin in tissues, and the accumulation of free iron ions, which generate tissue-damaging oxygen radicals. The consequences of hemochromatosis include enlargement of the liver; diabetes mellitus, as a result of radical damage to pancreatic β-islet cells (because of the skin pigmentation associated with hemochromatosis, the condition is sometimes called bronze diabetes); painful inflammation of joints; heart disease; and depletion of vitamin C, leading to scurvy.

One of the reasons why women are less at risk of atherosclerosis than are men may be that women generally have a lower iron status than men, because of menstrual blood losses. This raises the interesting problem of whether or not it is desirable to recommend high intakes of iron for women of child-bearing age in order to raise their iron reserves to the same level as seen in men. This would prevent the development of iron deficiency, but might also put them at risk of iron overload and increased risk of atherosclerosis.

5
Food and Nutrition

Classes of food–Proteins, starches and fats. Food furnish heat and energy for action and warmth.

All foods come from animals, vegetables or the air and water we take.

Animal foods include all meats, eggs, dairy foods and sea foods and are primarily proteins in their chemistry of promoting muscle action.

Vegetable foods are all leafy, root, tubers, nuts, grains, and are the foods that contain the highest vitality of all potential foods.

Minerals are found in both animal and vegetable kingdom and come from the soil, the water and when acted on by the sunshine, through the leaf of the plants, the minerals become carrier of vitality we have been taught to define as vitamins. The vitamins are the rejuvenators of cell life and minerals are the storage battery that carry the spark of life to the cells through the blood.

The essence of the science of nutrition is that the body needs a full and constant supply of minerals in balanced form, to know the science of nutrition is to know how to keep all cells properly fed so the level of cell life can be at its peak.

If there is a deficiency in food put into the blood stream through the digestive system, it is like using dead batteries or batteries that have lost their chargers of energy. Instead of living (the cells of the body that need energy die away).

The question of acidity or alkalinity is easy to answer. Minerals keep you alkaline and acids take minerals out of the body and therefore make you acid.

It is desirable to maintain a balance between acidity and alkalinity. Fruits, berries, sugars and acids have to be balanced with calcium, sodium, potassium, magnesium, iron and many other mineral elements. All fruits, including orange juice are of an acid nature and minerals are required in order to balance them. Milk is lactic acid in nature and actually softens bones and teeth.

Foods of the mineral kingdom are most important. But they must have the spark of life or they fall to energize cell life. Anti-life factors, such as anti-life drugs, insecticides, tranquillizers, stimulants and chemicals have not spark of life and, therefore, kill by degrees slowly, but surely. This killing process is the beginning of cancer and other known diseases. The eating of "dead food" causes the bowels to get lazy and decay takes place.

People have to be taught how to select and classify food so as to have a proper meal, a meal that will escape gastritis, acidity, headaches, heart pains and arthritis. We must learn to eat with balance.

Foods that cause trouble are sugars, acids and starches, as well as the sulphur foods such as cabbage, cauliflower, onions, radishes, leeks, turnips, mustard greens, broccoli, brussels-sprouts, watercress and egg yolks. Sulphur foods do not mix with any other class.

There are certain combinations of food that are desirable and others are undesirable. Here are some rules:

When Eating This Food	What To Eat Or Not Eat With Such Food
Meats, Sea foods, Eggs, Dairy	OK: Fresh fruits or green products and fowl. Salads of non-sulphur class. For salad dressing, use lime, lemon, oil and apple cider vinegar
Starches such as Rice	OK: Green salads. **NOT OK:** Fruit potatoes, grains, beans, or sugar or acid, puddings, muffins, pastries.
Cooked Vegetables	Salads of the same or any other fresh vegetable may be combined and eaten safely.
Sulphur foods	Eat no other class of foods with them except possibly a beverage of herbal tea without any sugar or sweetening.

In selecting food, obtain only organically grown foods that have not been sprayed. Every effort should be make to select meats free to chemicals. Only bread that is free of preservatives should be eaten and canned food should be avoided unless canned in a lacquered or keg-lined can or preserved in a glass container.

The following foods are undesirable for the reasons given:

Celery–bleached celery is old and devitalized.

Head lettuce–often treated with arsenic while growing.

White cabbage–often treated with arsenic while growing.

Apples–often full of absorbed arsenic from sprays.

Egg–dipped in chemicals during grading process. Chemicals go into eggs (toxic).

Cucumbers–covered with toxic and wax-like oil in stores.

Milk–so full of chemicals that usually it rots before it sours.

Ice creams, candies, carbonated water and gelatine desserts all loaded with carbolic acid by-products. (Cancerous, because of coal tar colours and flavours).

Balancing A Meal

If a concentrated protein is chosen for a meal, a light starch only should be combined with it. With this combination, a high mineral source food should be selected, or a mineral food supplement tablet.

If a moderate protein food is chosen, such as beans, peas, lentils, eggs or cheese, a medium starch can be combined advantageously and steamed vegetables of any type can be safely combined.

Never combine meats, flash, or fowl with leguminous, beans, and the concentrated dairy products, for one protein only suffices at a meal.

Eat green salads as a source of minerals and enzymes to promote the alkaline side of body balance.

Soups many be made in such a way as to comprise as balanced meal by itself.

The following instructions apply to making soups:

The Foundation–Put plenty of good vegetables into a glass or stainless steel pan of two to four quart size and cover the vegetables with an inch of water over the top of the level of the vegetables. However, avoid any of the sulphur vegetables (see Food and Nutrition). You may include plenty of parsley, celery, whole unpeeled potato, green string beans, green squash, chard, carrot tops, asparagus, artichokes, bell pepper and an egg in the shell. Salt to taste after the vegetables have been taken out of the pot. The liquid is saved as the foundation for adding of finely chopped green fresh vegetables just before serving. When removing the cooked vegetables from the pot or pan, save the egg and use it as a salad addition, for it will be hard-boiled and have more flavor by having been cooked in the broth.

The broth from the cooked vegetables can be used as a base for a wide variety of soup flavours.

For the most delicious creamed pea soup imaginable, take a package of fresh frozen green peas and place then into a quart of the broth and bring to a boil. Place into a liquifier for a minute or two and serve. Lentils may be soaked previously or cooked and also put into the broth. (A lentil is shaped about the same as a lens. The stem has leaves with 8 to 10 leaflets and has pale blue flowers. The pod is nearly as the legumes and may be used in any recipe that calls for dried beans). Barley may be added, fresh chopped celery, parsley and finely diced carrots added and simmered for a new seconds before serving.

Egg flower soup is made by adding Chinese cabbage, finely chopped, to the foundation broth with an egg stirred in while the broth is boiling.

Cream and tomato may be added to the broth for an unusual taste from it, to make all the vitamins in the food boil only to tenderize the food.

Meats should be boiled or barbecued and perhaps roasted, but slowly. Meat should never be fried or cooked in aluminium foil. Meat should be alkalinized in the cooking process and this is accomplished by the flame barbecue.

Waterless cooking in stainless steel containers is ideal as the flavour and the vitamins will be retained as well as the full natural colour. Vegetable may also be tenderized by lying the vegetables in parchment paper and immersing them in boiling water for 10 or 20 minutes. This way, they never reach a temperature over 180 degrees. To make vegetables for a salad crisp and firm, place into a large bowl and cover with a cup or two of chopped ice.

Pesticides–The book by Rachel Carson "Silent Spring" (Heughton Mifflin Company, Boston) explains in minute details the dangers of eating food that has been sprayed by pesticides. Miss Carson had a degree in biology and did graduate work in genetics and development. She was also in the employ of the United States Government as a biologist and editor, and she became world famous for her writings. She collected data from scientists all over the world about the dangerous effects of deadly poisons, especially in the form of synthetic insecticides, in the living community.

Many housewives feel that they can wash off certain poison sprays. What can be seen on the outside should be washed off, to be sure, but there is absorbed into the cells of the vegetables a high percentage of chemicals from soil and spray used by the grower. Even the fumes of insecticides generally present in a grocery store get into the exposed vegetables to some extent. In shopping for groceries, it is best not to shop in a store where fumes can be detected. It is well to ask the store manager what is used to kill bugs and flies, and whether or not the spraying is done under conditions when the spray may contact the vegetables.

Benzene has been recognized in medical literature for many years as a cause of leukaemia. Miss Carson points out that benzene is a frequent constituent of insecticidal solvents.

It lodges in the bone marrow and remains deposited there for periods known to be as long as 230 months.

Miss Carson writes: "Despite the warnings of cancer experts, carbamates are now widely used, not only as insecticides, weed killers, and fungicides, but also in a variety of products including plasticizers, medicines, clothing and insulating materials".

There is excessive exposure to cancer-producing chemicals, including pesticides. Quoting Miss Carson again: "An individual may have many different exposures to the same chemical. Arsenic is an example. It exist in the environment of every individual in many different guises: as an air pollutant, a contaminant of water a pesticide residue on food, in medicines, cosmetics, wood preservatives or as a colouring agent in paints in inks. It is quite possible that no one of these exposures alone would be sufficient to precipitate malignancy, yet any single supposedly "safe dose" may be enough to tip the scales that are already loaded with other "safe doses".

Thus, it is clear that while government reports may say that the amount of pesticides to be found upon vegetables or in the milk from cows grazing upon pesticide infected grasses is within the scope of a "safe dose", it must be borne in mind that there are other exposures in addition to the single exposure which the government has found to be safe. Furthermore, prolonged exposure to "safe doses" may result in a building up of the dangerous materials so as to become dangerous.

Pesticides have been proved to damage the liver and to reduce the supply of B vitamins, thus leading to an increase in the "endogenous" estrogens, or those produce by the body itself. Added to these are the wide variety of synthetic estrogens to which we are increasingly exposed. The combined effect is a matter that warrants the most serious concern. (From Miss Carson's book).

Oils–Lard and animal fats, coconut oil, oils in metals, oleomargarine and various other so-called vegetables shortenings are risky from the health standpoint. Natural oils that have not been heated or treated to prevent rencidity are the best. Sunflower seed oils and safflower seed oils are the very best.

Aluminium–Tests have revealed that aluminium cooking ware is unsafe because the food tends to absorb the aluminium from the aluminium metal. Also the use of aluminium foil is, for the same reason, to be avoided. Other synthetic coverings are also deleterious.

Organic Foods–In selecting food, every effort should be made to use organic foods, that is, foods grown without unnatural additives in the soil.

In selecting flavourings, select natural colouring and natural spices instead of chemicals and preservatives.

If non-organic food is used containing preservatives or grown with synthetic chemicals, tiny doses of poisons enter the body. The liver has to change these into bile and excrete or throw them off as best as it can. In time, these poisons affect the cells of the liver and the liver actually starts to break down and to harden and undergo cellular changes that produce symptoms such as gastritis, indigestion or acidosis, and allied results.

Among these poisons are included spray chemicals, coal tar, dyes, DDT, various other bug or germ killers, aspirin, anacin, phenobarbitol, sleeping pills, free metal found in cosmetics, free soft metals such as alum and double acting aluminium baking powders and many other substances that are inorganic chemicals used to preserve or colour food. These poisons accumulate in the body, usually at the weakest point, and lay the foundation for tissue breakdown and disease.

Meats–Meats should be boiled or barbecued. This eliminates frying, which is bad because the oil used is generally over-fried to the point where poisons are formed that become part of the meat and enters the body. Also in boiling, the soaking in the water results in valuable food elements leaving the meat and entering the water itself.

Vegetables–Vegetables should be cooked in glass containers or in stainless steel in order to avoid the danger of the metal entering the food. While tests indicate that the metal absorption occurs only to small degree. It must be remembered that whatever poison enters the system is combined with various other poisons from other sources. Therefore, it is important to prevent all poisons from entering the system.

Food combinations–Every meal should be planned to provide as early a complete combination of protein, carbohydrate and minerals as possible.

Soups–Soups are best when they are eaten alone. Soups dilute stomach acids and ferments and therefore, reduce the likelihood of other food being fully mixed with the digestive enzymes.

Berries–Berries and fresh fruits assist in the digestion of meats and heavy starches. The acid in fruits helps to digest meats. Good apple, cider vinegar also goes well with meals, if non-distilled, also lime or lemon juice. Canned fruits are not as desirable as fresh fruits, but canned blueberries, black berries, currents and some other similar fruits all help to digest meats.

Potatoes–The digestive requirements of the potato conflict with the requirements of meat and therefore, the heavy starchy potato should be reserved for the vegetable meals, such as plain salads or steamed vegetables.

Selection of Vegetables–The important necessity is obtaining vegetables with mineral content. For the highest concentration of minerals, people should select chard (variety of white beet, cultivated for the leaf), beet tops, spinach, parsley, turnips, romaine lettuce, squash, cucumbers, bell peppers, parsnips, peas, string beans, and other similar vegetables.

While certain synthetic iron compounds are available in drug stores that are supposed to furnish the body with iron, such iron preparations are either constipating or work the opposite way. But organic iron found in vegetable, which has gone through the metabolism of a plant, is utilized the best of all and rarely causes any gastrointestinal complications. (Quoting from "*Overfed but Undernourished*" by H. Curtis Wood, M.D. Exposition Press. New York). This author continues to say that other compounds needed by the body, such as copper, cobalt, iodine, manganese, etc. are best absorbed in the natural form.

Dr. Wood indicated that it is unlikely "that we can obtain the trace elements that we need even from a diet that is well-balanced and contains plenty of fresh vegetables". Further, he stated that food supplements are needed in order for the body to obtain all of the elements it needs. "Such organic mineral food supplements (kelp tablets) are safe, inexpensive, and may be of value in preventing some of the degenerative conditions that are so common with advancing years. Kelp tablets can be purchased at any health food store".

Analysis of one of the kelp tablets indicated the following elements to be present: Iodine, calcium, phosphorous, iron, copper, magnesium, manganese, sodium, potassium, chlorine, sulfur, barium, boron, chromium, lithium, nickel, silicon, silver, strontium, titanium, vanadium and zinc.

Desserts–Desserts need not be omitted from meals, provided that they are carefully chosen. They should be of low caloric nature and of a type that will not ferment. In fermentation, the organisms derive their nourishment from the original compound and yield products that are poisonous to be ferment. Fermentation causes when the nutrient is exhausted or when the product of fermentation is in excess of the nutrient. An excess quantity of food can ferment rapidly and cause the discomforts of gastritis and indigestion.

Powdered agar will not ferment. One level teaspoonful to a quart of water makes a lot of dessert. Boil for 10 minutes. Agar or plain gelatin, which is a pure protein, are both neutral in taste and may be used with all flavor fruits, as well as nuts, melons, berries, pineapple, banana, coconut, cranberries and similar items to make delicious desserts.

Food Habits

Food habits have been with us for a long time. They are as old as yesterday, as contemporary as today, as modern as tomorrow. Food habits are the response of individuals or groups to social and cultural pressures selecting, consuming, and utilization of proteins from the available food supply.

Food habits, the food-ways of cultures, are influenced by social organization. Through the study of habits of primitive tribes, it was found that the role of food was related to the social status as well as to the physical status of the members of the tribe. During pregnancy women are given favourite foods, the implication being that a prospective warrior might be born. Children were nourished from mothers breasts or from the milk of animals. The aged were nourished because they were the ones who could provide wisdom to the younger generation. However, in some tribes the aged were allowed to die, if they interfered with the activities of, or did not fulfil a useful function in the tribe. The strong, superior individuals helped to evolve a caste system. Those who did not make the upper grade of leadership were assigned to perform the necessary chores, to take care of the soil, crops and animals.

Today's social structure of rural and urban groupings has developed from yesterday's primitive tribes. In this country, since the beginning of the twentieth century, changes have occurred in social organization, with movement from rural to urban and metropolitan areas where factories are located. From the traditional slow pace of rural living, families have moved to city life where the tempo is accelerated by competitiveness. With the increasing urbanization in the United States during the past generation, breakfast and lunch have become skimpier and dinner larger. Except for rural areas where dinner is usually served at the noon meal, supper is rarely heard of. Authorities have questioned the advisability of the large dinner at night, which is usually followed by little or no physical activity.

Urban food supply included variety in food and variety in food service, while the characteristics of rural food supply are home grown products which are home-processed, home-cooked, and home served. However, present shipping centres throughout the country give urban and rural dwellers equal opportunities of choice in most sections of the United States. Ready to eat foods are available and utilized in both the urban and rural areas, thus replacing many of the home-prepared foods.

6
Nutrition, Diet & Development

During the first year, a baby grows and develops faster than any other time in life. The average baby measures from 18 to 22 inches in length at birth. A baby will grow about an inch per month for the first 6 months after birth. A baby who is 20 inches long at birth may be 30 inches long by his first birthday, about ½ time the length at birth.

A baby's birth weight will likely triple during the first year. A baby who weighs 7 pounds at the birth may weight approximately 21 pounds by the end of the first year. The vital organs of a baby's body grow rapidly, also brain weight doubles and the weight of the kidneys triples during this first year. The coming of teethe varies greatly from child to child.

The development of a baby's capabilities is also remarkable during the first year. A baby progresses from a newborn whose head must be supported while being feed, to a 6 month-old who may sit in a high-chair with little or no support, to a one year old who probably can drink from a cup with a bit of help.

All babies grow and develop at their own individual rate. No two babies are alike. There is a wide range of growth and activities that is considered normal.

The importance of good nutrition for a baby:

Everyone needs good nutrition throughout life to be healthy. Because of a baby's rapid growth, at no time is nutrition more important than during infancy. What a baby consumes must contain the proper nutrients in the right amounts to support the processes necessary for life.

Babies are not miniature adults, although they do have special needs because of their growth rate and immature body systems. Either too tittle or too much of the same nutrients can be balance of the right substance.

The nutrients needed by the baby are:

Proteins	Minerals
Carbohydrates	Vitamins
Fats	Water

These are found in varying amounts and foods both solid and liquid.

During the first year, particularly during the first 6 months, milk is a baby's primary food source. Human breast milk or infant formulas, which have been designed to be nutritionally as much like breast milk as possible, are most desirable for babies. Plain cow's milk has been found to represent unsuitable nutrition for a baby's first year.

The approximate calories per quart are:

1. Human Milk 700
2. Formula w/iron 643
3. Whole Cow's Milk 634
4. 2% Low Fat Milk 487
5. Skim Cow's Milk 343

Amounts of Calories in Milk Feedings

To grow and develop properly, babies need to consume about 50 calories every day for each pound that they weigh. For example a 10 pound baby needs about 500 calories each day. One fluid ounce of breast milk and one fluid ounce of formula have a similar number of calories (approx. 20 cal./OZ). So babies would need to consume about the same amount of these feedings to meet their caloric needs each day.

Whole cow's milk has a number of calories per fluid ounce, similar to breast milk and infant formula, but the proportions of fat, protein and carbohydrates are vastly different.

The number of calories in one fluid ounce of 2% low fat milk (approx. 15 cal/OZ) is only about three fourths as many calories as in the same quantity of breast milk or infant formula. Babies would need to drink more low fat cow's milk to get the calories they need for proper growth and activity.

There are only about half the number of calories in 1 OZ skim cow's milk as there are in breast milk or infant formula. Skim milk has approximately 11 calories per ounce. This means that babies would have to drink twice the amount of skim milk as they would not be able to tolerate such an amount to obtain the same calories they need.

Even with additional foods, the number of calories babies would consume in a day from drinking skim cow's milk would not be enough to allow for a normal growth. Skim cow's milk is not suitable as a milk feeding during infancy.

Nutrition in Childhood and Adolescence

Heredity and environment determine the way a child grows and the size and shape that he becomes. His genetic inheritance specifies how his bones will grow and what kind of a physique he will have. His environment during the period of growth when cells multiply and increase in size may encourage of inhabit genetic possibilities. Growth of the young reflect individual health. Adequate nutrition and freedom from diseases play important role in the determining whether an individual attains his potential. A disease disrupts normal growth patterns. Development that is, the changes in growth of an individual, is progressive and leads eventually to maturity. The rate (of age) at which growth and development takes place varies with each individual. The danger of accepting any "standard measurement" of growth and development and the tendency to hold too rigidly to exact figures. An individual must be assessed according to many factors attributing to his growth and development. The nutritional requirements, rational stage, physical activity, efficiency of healthy growth and development depends more on good nutrition than any other factor.

There are four phases of growth, they are:

Infancy–a period of very rapid growth.

Childhood–a period of slower but uniform growth.

Adolescence–a period of marked acceleration.

Post Adulthood–a period of gradual decline of growth until its cessation.

From the beginning of growth in the prenatal period to the time when a child attains his full size as an adult, the food that he eats and his ability to convert that food into energy and new body tissues will influence the state of his health not only as a child but throughout his whole life.

Excessive fat in the face is called as steatorrhoes. **Low fat diet includes:**

Cereals–200gms., Pulses–100gms., Leafy vegetables–100gms., Potato, Sugar, Banana–50gms., Orange–100gms., Ghee, Oil-cooked food–15gms., Chicken-Fish–100gms., Eggs–1, Milk–100ml. This diet provides 2100 Calories (Protein–75gms., Fat–30gms., Carbohydrates–385gms.).

Low Sodium Diet:

Normal diet with low sodium means, food cooked without additional salts. This is used in conditions of Oedema, Nephritis, Cardiac Diseases, Toxaemia of Pregnancy, hypertension.

Food cooked with salts, baking soda, pickles, nutmegs etc., should be avoided.

It includes Rice–250gms., Dal–100gms., Fruits and Vegetables–200, Milk–200ml., Oil, Sugar–50gms., Meat or Fish–50gms., Eggs–1. It provides 2,200 Calories (Protein–70gms., Sodium–0.5gms.).

Low Oxalic Acid Diet:

Patients suffering from oxaloacetic calculi should take low oxalic acid diet. It includes Rice, Wheat–200gms., Dal–5gms., Cabbage, Cauliflower–50gms., Mango–1, Potato–75gms., Milk–200ml., Oil, Sugar–30gms., Mutton, Egg–30gms.

It provides 2,400 Calories (Protein–65gms., Fat–50gms., CHO–425gms.).

More of leafy vegetables, and other vegetables must not be used like Brinjal, Beans, Onion, Stalks, Green Mango, Tomato, Ladies Finger etc., Tea, Coffee should not be used.

Cereals-300gms., Pulses-100gms., Leafy Vegetables 100gms., Roots, Sugar, Banana-50gms., Orange-100gms. Ghee, Oil-cooked food-15gms., Chicken-Fish-100gms. Egg-1, Milk-400ml. The diet provides 2400 Calories (Protein-70gms., Fat-40gms., Carbohydrate-385gms.)

Low Sodium Diet:

Normal diet with low sodium means food cooked without additional salt. This is used in conditions of Oedema, Nephritis, Cardiac Diseases, Toxaemia of Pregnancy, Hypertension.

Food cooked with salt, baking soda, pickles, namkeens etc. should be avoided.

It includes: Rice-350gms., Dal-100gms., Fruits and Vegetables-300, Milk-200ml., Oil, Sugar-50gms., Meat or Fish-50gms., Eggs-1. It provides 2,200 Calories (Protein-70gms., Sodium-0.5gms.)

Low Oxalic Acid Diet:

Patients suffering from oxaloacetic calculi should take low oxalic acid diet. It includes Rice, Wheat-300gms., Dal-75gms., Cabbage, Cauliflower-50gms., Mango-1, Potato-75gms., Milk-200ml, Oil, Sugar-40gms., Mutton, Egg-30gms.

It provides 2,500 Calories (Protein-65gms., Fat-50gms., CHO-425gms.)

More of leafy vegetables and other vegetables must not be used like Brinjal, Beans, Onion, Saika, Green Mango, Tomato, Ladies Finger etc., Tea, Coffee should not be used.

7
Nutrition & Diet Therapy

Nutrition- study of nutrients and the processes by which they are used by the body. It is the combination of processes by which the body utilizes food for growth, energy, and maintenance. It is concerned with the study of food and its relation to health and disease.

Malnutrition-results when the organism fails to receive or cannot utilize the essential nutrients.

Dietetics-is the application of the science of nutrition and food management to the feeding of individuals or groups.

The Dietician is particularly aware in the variation on nutrient needs determined by sex, age, activity, and physical condition of the individual or group. Psychology as well as socioeconomic factors plays an important role in the functions of the dietician.

Basic Concepts of Nutrition

1. Nutrition is the food you eat and how the body uses it. We eat food to live, to grow, to keep healthy and well, and to get energy for work and play.
2. Food is made up of different nutrients needed for growth and health.

a. All the nutrients needed by the body are available through food.

b. Many kinds and combination of food can lead to a well-balanced diet.

c. No food, by itself has all the nutrients needed for full growth and health.

d. Each nutrient has its specific uses in the body.

e. Most nutrients do their best work in the body when teamed with other nutrients.

3. All persons, throughout life, have need for the nutrients but in varying amounts

   a. The amounts of nutrients needed are influenced by age, sex, activity and the state of health.

   b. Suggestions for the kinds and amounts of food are made by trained scientist.

4. The way food is handled influences the amount of nutrients in food, its safety, appearance, and taste.

   a. Handling means everything that happen to food while it is being grown, processed, stored and prepared for eating.

Variables Affecting an Individual's Calorie Needs

1. Age and Growth
2. Gender
3. Climate
4. Sleep
5. Activity
6. Fever
7. Illness

Food and Fluid Intake Regulating Mechanisms

Hypothalamus

1. Thirst–triggered by loss of body fluid more than 2%
2. Hunger–triggered by low blood glucose level
3. Appetite–triggered by sight, smell, and thought of food
4. Satiety–triggered by gastric distension

Nurses' Role in Diet Therapy

A. Assess nutritional status
B. Observe nutritional intake
C. Evaluate response to diet therapy
D. Support dietary teaching and regimen ordered

The nurse plays and important part in the nutritional aspect of patient care.

Because of being close and continual contact with the patient, the nurse is able to evaluate the patient's nutritional status and provide input to the dietician about the patient's nutritional needs and acceptance of the nutritional plan of care.

Good nutrition is essential to good health throughout the life cycle and the nurse is an excellent position to encourage sound nutritional practice whenever possible in each patient encountered.

Clinical Signs of Nutritional Status

	Features	**Good**	**Bad**
1	General appearance	Alert, responsive	Listless, apathetic, cachexia
2	Hair	Shiny, lustrous, healthy scalp	Dull, brittle, dry, depigmented
3	Neck glands	No enlargement	Thyroid enlarged

	Features	Good	Bad
4	Skin, face, neck	Smooth, slightly moist, good color, reddish pink mucus membrane	Greasy, discoloured scaly
5	Eyes	Bright, clear, no fatigue circles	Dryness, increased vascularity, glassiness, thickened conjunctiva
6	Lips	Good color, moist	Dry, scaly, swollen, angular lesions (stomatitis)
7	Gums	Good pink color, no swelling or bleeding, firm	Marginal redness or swelling, receding, spongy
8	Tongue	Good pink color, surface papillae present, no lesion	Papillary atrophy, smooth appearance, swollen, red, beefy (glossitis)
9	Teeth	Straight, no crowding, well shaped jaw, clean, no discoloration	Unfilled cavities, absent teeth, worn surface, mottled, malpositioned
10	Skin, general	Smooth, slightly moist, good color	Rough, dry, scaly, pale, pigmented, irritated, petechiae, bruises
11	Abdomen	Flat	Swollen
12	Legs, feet	No tenderness, weakness, swelling, good color	Edema, tender calf, tingling, weakness

	Features	Good	Bad
13	Skeleton	No malformations	Bowlegs, knock-knees, chest deformity at diaphragm, beaded ribs, prominent scapulae
14	Weight	Normal for height, age, body build	
15	Posture	Erect, arms and legs straight, abd in, chest out	Sagging shoulders, sunken chest, humped back
16	Muscles	Well-developed. firm	Flaccid, poor tone, undeveloped, tender
17	Nervous control	Good attention span	Inattentive, irritable

Primary Causes of Nutritional Deficiency

1. Dietary lack of specific essential nutrients
   a. Lack of proper food
   b. Anorexia (due to a variety of causes)
   c. Alcoholism
   d. Poor food habits or eating nutritionally deficient foods
   e. Inadequate or faulty therapeutic diets
2. Inability of the body to use specific nutrient properly due to:
   a. Disease of the digestive tract such as ulcerative colitis
   b. Faulty absorption in intestinal tract (such as the way

in which the excessive use of mineral or impedes the absorption of fat-soluble vitamins)

c. Metabolic disorder such as diabetic

8
Nutrition for Infants, Children, Adults, Women and Elderly

Nutrition for Infants

2 Months

Baby will get all of his nutrition from breast milk or an iron fortified infant formula until he is four to six months old. There is no need to supplement with water, juice or cereal at this time. He should now be on a more predictable schedule and will probably be nursing or drinking 5-6 ounces of formula every 3-4 hours.

Feeding practices to avoid are putting the bottle in bed or propping the bottle while feeding, putting cereal in the bottle, feeding honey, introducing solids before 4-6 months, or heating bottles in the microwave.

Also, avoid the use of low iron formulas, which are nutritionally inadequate to meet the needs of a growing infant. These types of infant formula do not contain enough iron and will put your child at risk for developing iron deficiency anaemia (which has been strongly associated with poor growth and development and with learning disabilities). Iron fortified formulas do not cause colic, constipation or reflux and you should not switch to a low iron formula if your baby has one of these problems.

4 Months

At this age, breast milk or formula is the only food that your baby needs and he should be taking 5-6 ounces 4-6 times each day (24-32 ounces), but you can start to familiarize your baby with the feel of a spoon and introduce solid baby foods. See the Guide to Starting Solids for more information, especially if your child is at risk for developing food allergies.

Cereal is the first solid you should give your baby and you can mix it with breast milk, formula or water and feed it to your baby with a spoon (not in a bottle). Start by feeding one tablespoon of an iron-fortified Rice cereal at one feeding and then slowly increase the amount to 3-4 tablespoons one or two times each day. This is a very important source of iron for your growing infant (especially if you are breastfeeding). You can then start with vegetables at about six months of age.

Your baby will probably have given up middle of the night feedings by this age. If not, slowly reduce how much you are putting in the bottle each night and gradually stop this feeding all together. Feeding practices to avoid are putting the bottle in bed or propping the bottle while feeding, putting cereal in the bottle, feeding honey, using a low-iron formula or heating bottles in the microwave.

6 Months

While continuing to give 4-5 feedings of breast milk or formula (24-32 ounces) and 4 or more tablespoons of iron fortified cereal each day, you can now start to give well-cooked, strained, or mashed vegetables or commercially prepared baby foods. Start with one tablespoon of a mild tasting vegetable, such as green beans, peas, squash or carrots and gradually increase to 4-5 tablespoons one or two times each day.

Start fruits about a month after starting vegetables and again,gradually increase to 4-5 tablespoons one or two times each day. You can use peeled, cooked, or canned fruits (but only those packed in light syrup or water) that have been blenderized or strained.

You can also begin to offer 4-6 ounces of 100% fruit juices. Start by mixing one part juice with two parts of water and offer it in a cup only. Delay giving finger foods or meat and other protein foods until infants are eight to nine months old.

To avoid having to supplement with fluoride, prepare powdered/ concentrated formula with fluorinated tap water. If you are using ready to-feed formula, or bottled or filtered water only, then your baby may need fluoride supplements.

Your baby will probably have given up middle of the night feedings by this age. If not, slowly reduce how much you are putting in the bottle each night and gradually stop this feeding all together.

Feeding practices to avoid are putting the bottle in bed or propping the bottle while feeding, putting cereal in the bottle, feeding honey, using a low-iron formula, offering juice in a bottle or heating bottles in the microwave.

9 Months

While continuing to give 3-4 feedings of breast milk or formula (24-32 ounces) and 4 or more tablespoons of cereal, vegetables and fruit one or two times each day, you can now start to give more protein containing foods. These include well-cooked, strained or ground plain meats (chicken, beef, turkey, veal, lamb, boneless fish, or liver), mild cheese, peanut butter, or egg yolks (no egg whites as there is a high chance of allergic reactions in infants less than 12 months old).

If using commercially prepared jars of baby food, do not use vegetables with meat as they have little meat and less protein and iron than jars with plain meat.

Start with 1-2 tablespoons and increase to 3-4 tablespoons once each day. If your baby doesn't seem to like to eat plain meat, then you can mix it with a vegetable that they already like as you offer it.

You should start to offer soft table foods and finger foods at this age. Give soft, bite-size pieces of food, such as soft fruit and vegetable pieces, pastas, graham or saltine crackers, and dry cheerios, but do not give these foods if the child is going to be unattended in case of choking.

Over the next three months your baby's diet will begin to resemble that of the rest of the families, with 3 meals and 2 snacks each day. You can also give 4-6 ounces of 100% fruit juice in a cup.

To avoid having to supplement with fluoride, prepare powdered/concentrated formula with fluorinated tap water. If you are using ready to-feed formula, or bottled or filtered water only, then your baby may need fluoride supplements.

Your baby will probably have given up middle of the night feedings by this age. If not, slowly reduce how much you are putting in the bottle each night and gradually stop this feeding all together.

Feeding practices to avoid are changing to regular milk before your child is twelve months old, putting the bottle in bed or propping the bottle while feeding, feeding honey, using a low-iron formula, offering juice in a bottle or heating bottles in the microwave.

12 Months

You may now give your baby homogenized whole cow's milk. 2%, low fat, or skim milk are not recommended until your child is 2-3 years old. Your baby's diet will begin to resemble that of the rest of the families, with 3 meals and 2 snacks each day.

You should limit milk and dairy products to about 16-24oz each day (in a cup or bottle) and juice to 4-6 oz each day (offered in a cup only) and offer a variety of foods to encourage good eating habits later.

Your child should want to feed himself with his fingers and a spoon or fork and should be able to drink out of a cup.

The next few months will be time to stop using a bottle. Remember that your baby's appetite may decrease and become pickier over the next few years as his growth rate slows.

Your baby will probably have given up middle of the night feedings by this age.

If not, slowly reduce how much you are putting in the bottle each night and gradually stop this feeding all together.

If you are using bottled or filtered water only, then your child may need fluoride supplements .

Feeding practices to avoid are giving large amounts of sweet desserts, soft drinks, fruit-flavored drinks, sugarcoated cereals, chips or candy, as they have little nutritional value. Also avoid giving foods that your child can choke on, such as raw carrots, peanuts, whole grapes, tough meats, popcorn, chewing gum or hard candy.

Nutrition for Young Children

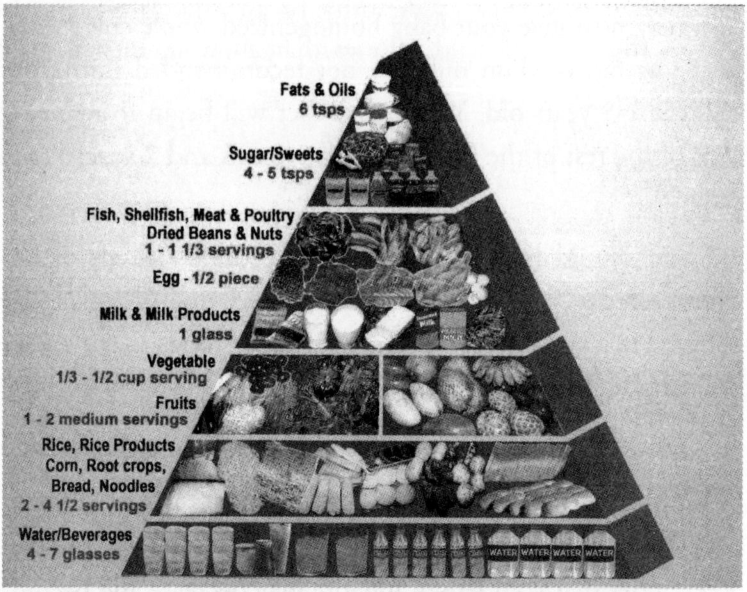

Fig.: Nutrition Pyramid for Young Children

In the first year of life, infants undergo periods of rapid growth when a good diet is crucial. In fact, nutrition in the early years of life is a major determinant of healthy growth and development throughout childhood and of good health in adulthood. Pediatricians and nutritionists have established nutritional guidelines to meet the specific needs of these early years. While there is great variety in the types of foods each infant and young child will gradually add to his or her diet, some generalizations may be helpful. If you are at all unsure about what or how to feed your infant during the first year of life, consult with your healthcare provider.

Breast milk is the ideal food for infants during the first six months of life. It contains still-undiscovered substances that cannot be reproduced artificially and its overall nutrient composition is superior to any alternative, including infant formula. In spite of its superiority, breast milk cannot provide all of the nutrients and calories that allow infants to thrive after the first six months of life. All infants should continue to receive breast milk for at least the first year and preferably for the second, but other, more nutritious foods should be added by the time an infant reaches six months of age. Formula-fed infants usually require only formula for their first year, but they should also be introduced to other kinds of foods once they reach six months of age.

From the age of six months until approximately two years, infants and young children should gradually be introduced to different types of semi-solid, solid or complementary foods as they gradually transition from a diet centered on breast milk or formula. This transition period helps the child to slowly become accustomed to eating adult-type foods and familiarizes them with a wide range of textures and tastes.

Most infants begin the transition from liquid to solid foods with the introduction of infant cereals. When mixed with breast milk or formula, cereal can be a good starting place. Eating cereals from a spoon takes practice, but most 6-month olds are able to adapt quickly. After introducing cereal, many mothers next begin offering pureed or mashed vegetables and fruits. Whether prepared industrially or at home, these foods are a pleasant introduction to new tastes and textures. Gradually, the smooth, pureed foods can be replaced with foods of more solid texture, such as meat or fish based meals, until the infant begins to eat table food. Introducing your infant to complementary foods is a gradual and, at times, trying process. The key to success is to gradually move from fairly bland and smooth foods to foods that are more robust in texture, taste, and smell. Be creative in planning meals and have fun, this exciting and challenging stage will surely produce many rare memories.

Commercial Foods

Many so called prepared complementary foods are available to help your infant make the transition from breast milk or formula to solid food. While some parents choose to prepare their own foods, others find that industrially prepared foods are convenient, safe, and nutritious alternatives.

Commercial foods are formulated to satisfy the nutritional needs of infants and young children. These are mainly sold in dried form and need reconstituting by adding water or milk. Meat, vegetables and fruit are major ingredients, these may be given mixed with cereals, cornflakes, oats, semolina or pasta. There are also a whole of biscuits, rusks, protein and chocolate bars to desserts and drinks available to choose.

Commercial Foods are ready to eat baby foods; these consist of prepared recipes that are cooked and sterilized and are normally sold in cans and jars. This broad category includes baby meals, fruit or vegetable based foods, and meat and fish based foods.

Dried baby foods; the range of dried foods available is similar to ready-to-eat and they are prepared according to recipes, but they are dried after cooking. Dried foods must be mixed with water or milk before feeding.

Cereal-based foods; these are usually sold dried and ready for reconstitution. They are based on pre-cooked cereals with additions of meat, vegetables or fruit. Some are reconstituted with milk, but others are already mixed with high protein foods and should be reconstituted with a non-protein containing liquid such as water.

Pasta; these are available with different shapes and are used after cooking in boiling water or other appropriate liquid.

Biscuits and rusks; these can be offered in dried form or can be soaked in water or milk. These products can be particularly useful for teething infants.

Milk based desserts; special deserts with controlled sugar content typically contain yogurt or other milk products as a main ingredient.

Flavoured Milk; special formulations of cow's milk or soy extracts have been developed to match the specific nutritional needs of young children over one year of age.

Other drinks; these may be convenient to feed infants and are specially formulated as an introduction to the texture of adult foods while meeting the strict dietary requirements of infants and young children. Their manufacturers ensure they are processed according to the strictest hygiene and safety requirements as well as formulated to meet nutritional standards established by health authorities throughout the world.

Whether you are giving your child homemade foods or commercially prepared foods, remember to keep your child's diet varied and appropriate to his or her stage of development. The inappropriate use of adult foods may result in insufficient intake of some nutrients, such as iron and fat, or an excess of others, such as salt and fibre. Stay with foods meant for infants at first and then gradually introduce foods meant for adults . Fruit, vegetable and herbal drinks also contain controlled amounts of sugar. Although all infants require a liquid diet during the first months of life, solid foods eventually become the predominant source of nutrition. No infant should be introduced to solid or complementary foods before the age of four months and, in many cases, it may be better to wait until the infant is at least six months old.

By six months of age, your infant's nutritional needs are beginning to increase. Breast milk or infant formula, alone, may not provide all the nutrients your infant needs to continue growing and developing. The purpose of introducing complementary foods is to provide a more energy- dense diet with adequate protein for growth and a high proportion of calories from fat. In addition, commercial or home made foods are a good way to introduce new tastes and textures so your infant can eventually graduate to eating the same meals as the rest of your family.

In the past, many mothers started feeding solid foods too early, before their baby's digestive organs were sufficiently developed. In addition, semi-solid foods must be fed with a small spoon. Yet, before the age of four to six months, the infant's nervous system is not sufficiently developed to allow use of a spoon. Before starting to eat solid foods, your infant should be able to sit easily with support and coordinate chewing and swallowing. Solid foods such as cereal should never be placed in a bottle for feeding.

When starting the transition to complementary foods, milk or an appropriate formula should continue to be a major part of the infant's diet. Whole cow's milk or goat's milk, which are widely used by mothers throughout the world, are not appropriate as an exclusive source of food for infants. For this reason, and at the request of the medical profession, follow-on formulas were developed to meet the nutritional needs of older infants. They provide the liquid part of a weaning diet and, because they contain more iron, more vitamin D and less saturated fat, are nutritionally more appropriate than whole cow's milk or other animal milks.

Safety of Baby Foods

Commercial baby foods are made according to the highest microbiological and nutritional specifications and all ingredients must meet strict safety and quality standards. Thorough heat treatment, combined with strict hygiene standards, ensures the sterility of the product throughout the manufacturing process. The protein content of commercial baby foods varies, usually, baby foods contain less non-veg protein than other protein products do. Large amounts of non-veg protein can be overpowering for babies in terms of taste, smell and texture. Consequently, manufacturers try to balance the ingredients in protein-based baby foods to ensure palatability and good nutrition. The protein content and protein quality of baby foods are far more important than actual protein content.

Thus, manufacturers control the total amount of protein (which may include animal protein) in their products to supply enough for optimal growth and development of infants without straining their kidneys. They also pay attention to the mixture of amino acids in baby foods by using a variety of protein sources including meat, fish, milk, eggs, vegetables and cereals. As a standard practice, manufacturers provide labels showing the percentage of animal protein contained in all sachets and packets of commercial baby foods. Manufacturers cannot claim that individual foods are 'organic' unless an accredited body, has certified that the ingredients comply with specific standards. The most well-known organic standard is the restriction on the use of artificial fertilisers and pesticides, which protects most organic foods from containing pesticide residues.

Due to legislations, all baby foods are subject to very strict controls on pesticide residues as the law requires the level of any pesticides to be below 10 parts per billion. Whether the foods are labeled organic or not, artificial preservatives, colourings, sweeteners and artificial flavourings cannot be used in baby foods.

Nutrition for School-age Children

Child's nutrition is important to her overall health. Proper nutrition can also prevent many medical problems, including becoming overweight, developing weak bones, and developing diabetes. It will also ensure that your child physically grows to her full potential.

The best nutrition advise to keep your adolescent healthy includes encouraging her to; eat a variety of foods, balance the food you eat with physical activity, choose a diet with plenty of grain products, vegetables and fruits, choose a diet low in fat, saturated fat, and cholesterol, choose a diet moderate in sugars and salt, choose a diet that provides enough calcium and iron to meet their growing body's requirements. Healthy eating habits and regular exercise should be a regular part of your family's life. It is much easier if everyone in the house follows these guidelines, than if your child has to do it alone. You should also buy low-calorie and low fat meals, snacks and desserts, low fat or skim milk and diet drinks. Avoid buying high calorie desserts or snacks, such as snack chips, regular soft drinks or regular ice cream.

The Food Pyramid has been designed to promote healthy nutrition in children over two years of age. It is meant to be a general guide to daily food choices. The main emphasis of the Food Guide Pyramid is on the five major food groups, all of which are required for good health. It also emphasizes that foods that include a lot of fats, oils and sweets should be used very sparingly.

The Food Pyramid shows a range of servings for each food group. How much you actually eat depends on your age and activity level. School-age children require about 1600 to 2400 calories each day, depending on their age and activity level. Once they hit their growth spurt, girls require an additional 200 calories and boys 500 calories. School age children will therefore require between the low and middle range of servings. Children who are overweight and dieting should at least eat the lowest range of servings.

When determining how many servings to eat, it is important to look at the serving size. Larger portions should count as more than one serving, and smaller portions will count as only a part of a serving.

Fats, Oils and Sweets in Food

No more than 30% of your child's diet should come from fats. For a 1600 calorie diet, that would equal 53g of fat each day and for a 2200 calorie diet, 73g of fat each day.

The type of fat that your child eat is also important. Saturated fats in foods such as meats, dairy products, coconut, palm and palm kernal oil, raise cholesterol more than unsaturated fats, which are found in olive, peanut, and canola oils, or polyunsaturated fats in safflower, sunflower, corn, soybean and cottonseed oils. Limit saturated fats to no more than 10% of daily calories.

Sugars supply a large amount of calories, with little nutritional value. They include white sugar, brown sugar, corn syrup, honey and molasses and foods like candy, soft drinks, jams, and jellies.

Use lean meats and low fat dairy products. Limit foods that contain a large amount of saturated fats and sugar.

Food	Servings	Grams of Fat
Butter, margarine	1 tsp.	04
Mayonnaise	1 tbs.	11
Salad dressing	1 tbs.	7
Sour cream	2 tbs.	6
Cream cheese	1 oz.	10
Chocolate bar	1 oz.	9

Milk, Yogurt and Cheese

Dairy products provide protein, vitamins and minerals and are an excellent source of calcium. Your schoolage child should have 2 to 3 servings of milk, yogurt and cheese each day. Choose skim milk and non-fat yogurt. Avoid high fat cheese and ice cream.

Food	Servings	Grams of Fat
Skim milk, 1 cue	1	Trace Non-fat
Yogurt, 8 oz	1	Trace
Lowfat milk, 1 cue	1	5
Whole milk, 1 cue	1	8
Chocolate milk, 2%, 1 cue	1	5
Lowfat yougurt, 1 cue	1	4
Process cheese, 2 oz.	1	18
Mozzarella, Eart skin 1-1/2 oz	1	7
Cottage cheese, 1/2 cue	1/4	5
Ice cream, 1/2 cue	1/3	7
Ice milk, 1/2 cue	1/3	3
Frozen rogurt, 1/2 cue	1/2	2

Meat, Poultry, Fish, Dry Beans, Eggs and Nuts

Foods in this group provide protein, vitamins and minerals, including B vitamins, iron and zinc. You should give 2 to 3 servings of foods from this group each day, including the equivalent of 5 to 7 ounces of lean meat. A serving from this food group can include 2-3 ounces of lean meat, poultry or fish, which may be an average hamburger or medium chicken breast half , and dry beans and peas. Prepare meats by trimming away fat, and broiling, roasting, or boiling rather than frying. Remember that nuts and seed are high in fat, and egg yolks are high in cholesterol, so you should eat them in moderation.

Food	Servings	Grams of Fat
Lean meat, Poultry, fish	30z	6
Ground beef, lean	30z	16
Chicken, with skin, fried	30z	13
Bologna, 2 slices	10z	16
E!2g, 1	10z	5
Dry beans and Peas, 1/2 cup	10z	Trace
Peanut butter, 2 tbs.	10z	16
Nuts, 1/3 cup	10z	22

Vegetables

Vegetables supply your child with vitamins, including vitamin A and C, and folate, minerals, such as iron and magnesium, and fibre. Plus they are low in fat. You should have 2 to 4 servings of vegetables each day. You should eat a variety of vegetables to provide you with all of the different nutrients that they supply, including dark green leafy vegetables, deep yellow vegetables, starchy vegetables (potatoes, corn peas), legumes (navy, pinto and kidney beans), and other vegetables (lettuce, tomatoes, onions, green beans). Do not add a lot of fat to the vegetables by adding extra toppings, such as butter, mayonnaise, and salad dressings.

Food	Servings	Grams of Fat
Vegs, cooked, 1/2 cup	1	Trace
Vegs, leafy, raw 1 cup	1	Trace
Vegs, nonleafy, raw, 1/2 cup	1	Trace
Potatoes, scalloped, 1/2 cup	1	4
Potato salad, 1/2 cup	1	8
French fries, 10	1	8

Fruits

Fruits and 100% natural fruit juices provide Vitamin A and C and potassium. They are also low in fat and sodium. Your child should have 2-4 servings of fruit each day. Give fresh fruits and 100 % natural fruit juices and avoid canned fruits loaded with syrups and sweeteners. Give whole fruits, citrus fruits, melons, and berries, which are high in Vitamin C.

Food	Servings	Grams of Fat
Whole fruit	1	Trace
Fruit, raw or canned, 1/2 cup	1	Trace
Fruit juice, unsweetened, 3/4 cup	1	Trace
Avocado, 1/4 whole	1	9

Bread, Cereal, Rice and Pasta

Foods from this group provide complex carbohydrates (starches) and provide vitamins, minerals, and fibre. Your child needs at least 6 to 11 servings of foods from this food group each day. Choose whole grain breads and cereals for added fibre. Choose foods that are low in fat and sugars. Avoid adding calories and fat to foods in this group by not adding spreads or toppings high in fat.

Food	Servings	Grams of Fat
Bread, 1 slice	1	1
Hamburger roll	2	2
Tortilla	1	3
Rice, pasta, 1/2 cup	1	Trace
Breakfast cereals, 1 oz	1	?
Pancakes, 2	2	3
Croissant, 1 large	2	12
Doughnut, 1 medium	2	11
Danish, 1 medium	2	13
Cake, frosted, 1 slice	1	13
Cookies, 2 medium	1	4

Calcium Requirements

Calcium is a mineral that is mostly present in your child's bones. Having a diet with foods that are high in calcium to meet daily requirements is necessary for the development of strong bones. It is also an important way to prevent the development of osteoporosis in adults.

School-age children require about 800 mg of calcium each day. Once they reach puberty, their calcium requirements will increase to about 1200 mg each day. See the table for the calcium content of common foods and check the nutrition label to choose foods high in calcium when you prepare your families diet. Also choose foods that are rich in calcium.

Food	Servings	Calcium Content
Milk, whole or lowfat	1 cup	300 mg
White beans	1/2 cup	113 mg
Broccoli, cooked	1/2 cup	35 mg
Broccoli, raw	1 cup	35 mg
Cheddar cheese	1.5 oz	300 mg
Yogurt, lowfat	80z	300 mg
Orange juice, calcium fortified	1 cup	300 mg
Orange, medium	1	40-50 mg
Sweet potatoes, mashed	1/2 cup	mg

Iron Requirements

Iron is another mineral that is important for your child's growth. Having a diet with foods that are high in iron to meet daily requirements is necessary for the development of strong muscles and production of blood.

Adolescents require about 10 to 12 mg of iron each day. See the table for the iron content of common foods and check the nutrition label to choose foods high in iron when you prepare your families diet. Also choose foods that are fortified with iron (cereals, bread, rice, and pasta, etc.) and rich in iron like; beef, chicken, fish, liver, peanut butter, nuts and seeds, green peas, lima beans, pinto beans, spinach, greens, turnip/ collard, strawberries, tomato juice, squash, whole grain bread, raisins, watermelon, etc.

Nutrition for Adolescent

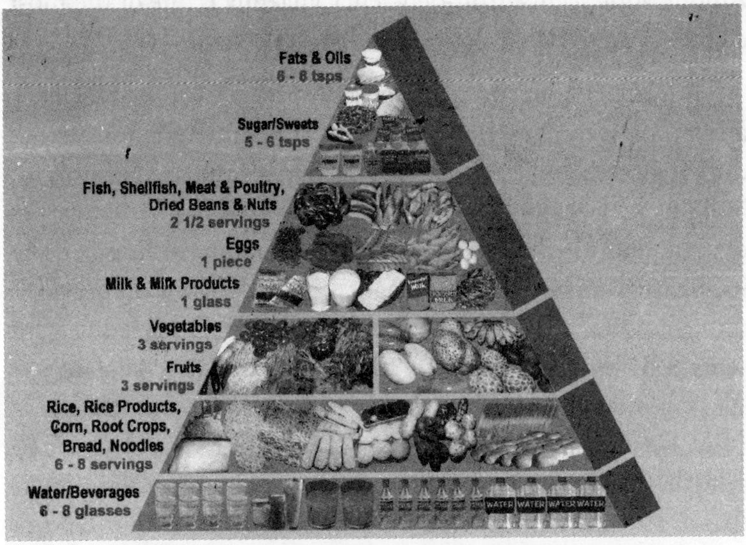

Fig.: Nutrition Pyramid for Adolescent

To develop to their optimal potential, it is vital that children are provided with nutritionally sound diets. Diet and exercise patterns during childhood and adolescence may spell the difference between health and risk of disease in later years. Different stages of the life cycle dictate differing nutrient needs.

The nutritional requirements of young people are influenced primarily by the spurt of growth that occurs at puberty. The peak of growth is generally between 11 and 15 years for girls and 13 and 16 years for boys. The nutrient needs of individual teenagers differ greatly, and food intake can vary enormously from day to day, so that those with deficient or excessive intakes on one day may well compensate on the next. In this period of life, several nutrients are at greater deficiency risk including iron and calcium.

Iron

Among adolescents, iron-deficiency anaemia is one of the most common diet-related deficiency diseases.

Adolescents are particularly susceptible to iron deficiency anaemia in view of their increased blood volume and muscle mass during growth and development. This raises the need of iron for building up haemoglobin, the red pigment in blood that carries oxygen, and for the related protein myoglobin, in muscle. The increase in lean body mass (LBM),composed mainly of muscle, is more important in adolescent boys than in girls. In preadolescent years, LBMis about the same for both sexes. Once adolescence starts, however, the boy undergoes a more rapid accumulation of LBM for each additional kilogram of body weight gained during growth, ending up with a final LBM maximum value double that of the girl. Other factors contributing to elevated iron needs are increased body weight and the beginning of menstruation for girls. All these factors should be taken into account when assessing iron needs in this group of age.

One of the most important diet considerations during adolescence is an increase in the intake of iron-rich foods such as lean meats and fish as well as beans, dark green vegetables, nuts and iron-fortified cereals and other grains. Iron from animal foods (known as haem iron) is much better absorbed than iron from non-animal sources (non-haem iron). Adolescents following vegetarian diets are therefore at an increased risk of iron deficiency. However, vitamin C (e.g., from citrus fruits) and animal proteins (meat, egg & fish) assist in the absorption of non-haem iron.

Calcium

The skeleton accounts for at least 99% of the body stores of calcium and the gain in skeletal weight is most rapid during the adolescent growth spurt. About 45% of the adult skeletal mass is formed during adolescence, although its growth continues well beyond the adolescent period and into the third decade. All the calcium for the growth of the skeleton must be derived from the diet. The largest gains are made in early adolescence, between about 10-14years in girls and 12-16years in boys.

During peak adolescent growth, calcium retention is, on average, about 200mg/day in girls and 300mg/day in boys. The efficiency of calcium absorption is only around 30% so it is important that the diet supplies an adequate calcium intake to help build the densest bones possible. The achievement of peak bone mass during childhood and adolescence is crucial to reduce the risk of osteoporosis in later years. By eating several servings of dairy products, such as milk, yoghurt and cheese, the recommended calcium intake can be achieved.

As well as a good dietary supply of calcium, other vitamins or minerals, like vitamin D and phosphorous, are needed for building up bones. Physical activity is also essential, particularly weight-bearing exercise, which provides the stimulus to build and retain bone in the body. Activities such as cycling, gymnastics, skating, ball games, dancing and supervised weight training for at least 30-60 minutes a day, three to five times a week can help build bone mass and density. Making the right dietary and lifestyle choices early in life will help young people develop health-promoting behaviours that they can follow throughout life.

Dietary habits, which affect food preferences, energy consumption and nutrient intakes, are generally developed in early childhood and particularly during adolescence. The home and school environments play a major role in determining a child's attitude to, and consumption of individual foods.

Teenagers, as well as being exposed to periodic food fads and slimming trends, tend to skip meals and develop irregular eating habits. One of the most frequently missed meal is breakfast. Studies suggest that breakfast plays an important role in providing needed energy and nutrients after an overnight fast and can aid in concentration and performance at school.

Snacks generally form an integral part of meal patterns for both children and teenagers. Younger children cannot eat large quantities at one sitting and often get hungry long before the next regular mealtime. Mid-morning and mid-afternoon snacks can help to meet energy needs throughout the day. Fast-growing and active teenagers often have substantial energy and nutrition needs and the teaching of food and nutrition in the school curricula will enable children to have the knowledge to make informed choices about the foods in their regular meals and snacks. Lack of activity plays an important role in the development, progression and perpetuation of obesity in adolescence. Surveys of young people have found that the majority is largely inactive and health professionals and governments are now encouraging higher levels of physical activity among children and adolescents. Physical inactivity does not only have a prime role in the development of overweight and obesity, but also on the development of chronic diseases such as heart disease, certain cancers, diabetes, hypertension, bowel problems and osteoporosis in later life. **In** addition, physical activity is related to improvements in body flexibility, balance, agility and co-ordination and strengthening of bones. The current recommendation is for children to try to be physically active for at least 60 minutes daily.

Nutrition for Adults

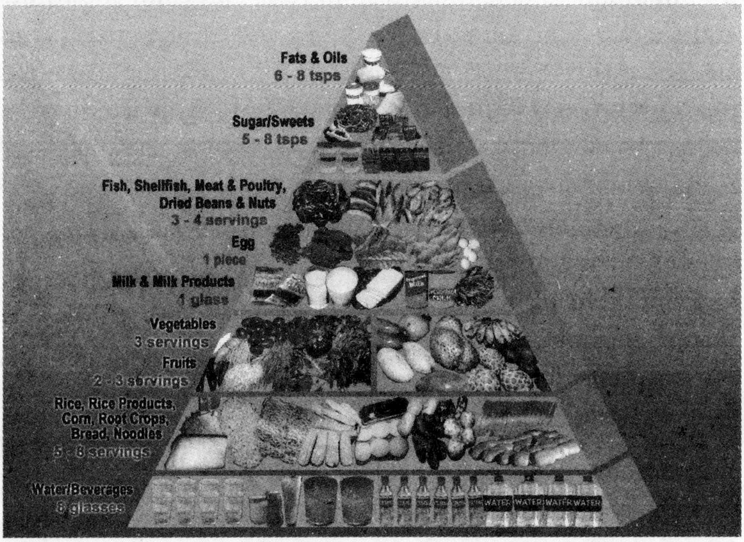

Fig.: Nutrition Pyramid for Adults

Healthy eating and a healthful way of life are important to how we look, feel and how much we enjoy life. The right lifestyle decisions, with a routine of good food and regular exercise, can help us make the most of what life has to offer. Making smart food choices early in life and through adulthood can also help reduce the risk of certain conditions such as obesity, heart disease, hypertension, diabetes, certain cancers and osteoporosis. Adults need wide variety viz., more than 40 different nutrients for good health and no single food can supply them all. So, consumption of a wide variety of foods (including fruits, vegetables, cereals and grains, meats, fish and poultry, dairy products and fats and oils), is necessary for good health and any food can be enjoyed as part of a healthy diet. Some studies have linked dietary variety with longevity. In any event, choosing a variety of foods adds to the enjoyment of meals and snacks. Eating is one of the life's great pleasures and it's important to take time to stop, relax and enjoy mealtimes and snacks. Scheduling eating times also ensures that meals are not missed, resulting in missed nutrients that are often not compensated for by subsequent meals. This is especially important for school children, adolescents and the elderly. Breakfast is particularly important as it helps kick-start the body by supplying energy after the all-night fast.

Balancing a meal means getting enough, but not too much, of each type of nutrient. If portion sizes are kept reasonable, there is no need to eliminate favourite foods. There are no 'good' or 'bad' foods, only good or bad diets. Any food can fit into a healthy lifestyle by remembering moderation and balance. Moderate amounts of all foods can help ensure that energy (calories) intake is controlled and that excessive amounts of anyone food or food component are not eaten. If you opt for a high fat meal, choose a lower fat option next time.

A healthy weight varies between individuals and depends on many factors including gender, height, age and hereditary.

Excess body fat results when more calories are eaten than are needed. Those extra calories can come from any source - protein, fat, carbohydrate or alcohol - but fat is the most concentrated source of calories. Physical activity is a good way of increasing the energy (calories) expended and it can also lead to feelings of well-being. It's quite simple, if you are gaining weight eat less and be more physically active.

Fruits and Vegetables

Numerous studies have shown an association between the intake of these foods and a decreased risk of cardiovascular disease and certain cancers. An increased intake of fruits and vegetables has also been associated with decreased blood pressure. People can fill up on fresh fruit and vegetables because they are good sources of nutrients and the majority are naturally low in fat and calories. Nutritionists are paying much more attention to fruits and vegetables and other constituents that are healthful for humans. Most antioxidants are found in fruits and vegetables like vitamins C and E , micronutrients as well as a number of other natural protective substances. The carotenes (beta-carotene, lutein and lycopene), the flavonoids (phenolic compounds that are widespread in commonly consumed fruits and vegetables such as apples and onions and beverages derived from plants like green tea, cocoa and red wine) and the phytoestrogens (chiefly isoflavones and lignans), are being propagated having beneficial roles in human health.

Most dietary guidelines recommend a daily diet in which at least 55% of the total calories should come from carbohydrates. This means making more than half of our daily food intake should consist of carbohydrate containing foods such as grains, pulses, beans, fruits, vegetables and sugars.

Although the body treats all carbohydrates in the same way regardless of their source, carbohydrates are often split into 'complex' and 'simple' carbohydrates. Complex carbohydrates that come from plants are called starch and fibres, and these are found for example in cereal grains, vegetables, breads, seeds, legumes and beans. These carbohydrates consist of long strands of many simple carbohydrates linked together. Simple carbohydrates (sometimes called simple sugars) are found for example in table sugar, fruits, sweets, jams, soft drinks, fruit juices, honey, jellies and syrups. Both complex and simple carbohydrates provide the same amount of energy (4 calories per gram) and both can contribute to tooth decay, especially when oral hygiene is not maintained properly.

Adults need to drink at least 1.5 litres of fluid daily, even more if it's hot for those are physically active. Plain water is a good source of liquid but variety can be both pleasant and healthy. Choose alternative fluids from juices, soft drinks, tea, coffee and milk.

Fat is a nutrient in food that is essential for good health. Fats provide a ready source of energy and enable the body to absorb, circulate and store the fat-soluble vitamins A, D, E and K. Fat-containing foods are needed to supply 'essential fatty acids' that the body cannot produce. Too much fat however, especially saturated fats, can lead to adverse health effects such as overweight and high cholesterol and increase the risk of heart disease and some cancers, by limiting the amount of fat, especially saturated fat in the diet -but not cutting it out entirely- is the best advice for a healthy diet. Most dietary recommendations are that less than 30% of the day's total calories should come from fat and less than 10% of the day's total calories should come from saturated fat.

The Salt Intake

Salt (NaCl) is made up of sodium and chloride. Sodium is a nutrient and is present naturally in many foods. Sodium and chloride are important in helping the body to maintain fluid balance and to regulate blood pressure. For most people, any excess sodium passes straight through the body however in some people it can increase blood pressure. Reducing the amount of salt in the diet of those who are sensitive to salt may reduce the risk of high blood pressure. However, the relationship between salt intake and blood pressure is still not known well and individuals should consult their doctor for advice.

Health Hazards of Unplanned Diet

Eating a lot without taking enough exercise can lead to weight gain and, ultimately, obesity.

With obesity comes a substantially increased risk of diabetes, cardiovascular disease, high blood pressure, some cancers and osteoarthritis. There is a lot of evidence to suggest that diets low in fruits, vegetables and pulses are associated with an increased risk of cancer and heart disease.

High salt consumption is linked to increased blood pressure and this is a risk factor for coronary heart disease. Saturated fats are the main dietary factor in increased blood cholesterol. 61% of men and 65% of women had raised cholesterol at levels linked with a higher risk of cardiovascular disease.

Frequent consumption of foods high in sugars increases the risk of tooth decay.

Nutrition for Pregnant & Lactating Women

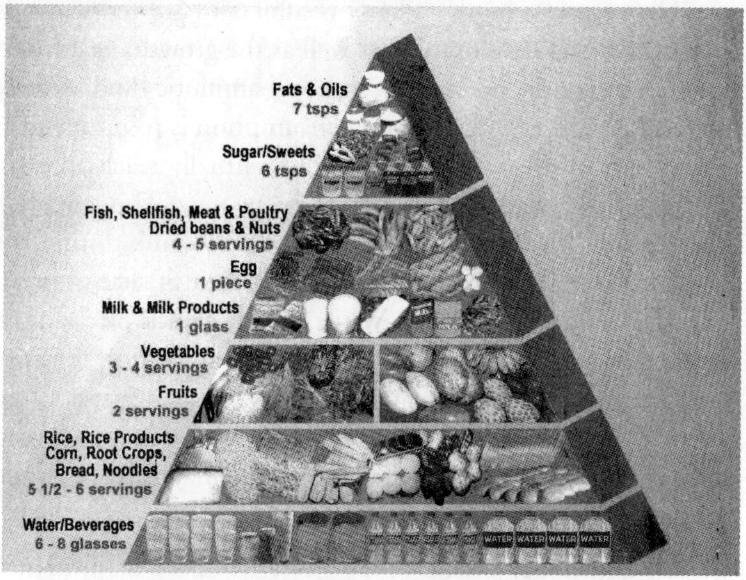

Fig: Nutrition Pyramid for Pregnant Women

Nutrition during pregnancy is important. Pregnant women's food has an affect on the pregnancy, on the fetal development and also on the health of the mother and child.

The foods a pregnant woman eat are the main source of the nutrients for the baby. It is important for pregnant women to understand what kind of food is best for them and their unborn baby, and a lactating women for her newborn.

A pregnant woman's nutrition directly influences the course of the pregnancy and normal fetal development, and also the long-term health of the mother and child. In the first half of pregnancy, nutrition requirements mainly concern quality, while in the second half, quantity is also an issue, to ensure fetal growth. Proper nutritional habits should already be established at the start of this second life ; if possible even before conception.

The pregnant mother's body is subject to greater demands to ensure foetal development as well as the growth, health and functioning of the uterus, placenta and amniotic fluid. A daily increase of 150 calories in food consumption is recommended at the start of pregnancy, which will eventually reach an extra 250 calories a day by the end of pregnancy. This entails a 'double-shot' in the form of a daily glass of milk during the first trimester and an additional piece of fruit or slice of bread during the final six months. While weight gain is normal, the mother-to-be should not let herself starting ,eating for two' (or more). The average weight gained is between 9 and 12 kg (20 to 26 lbs), although there is a natural variation between individuals. With overweight women, it may be less, while thinner women may gain more.

An additional intake of 10 g (1/3 ounce) of protein a day during the entire pregnancy is recommended to build up, maintain, and regenerate body tissue in both the fetus and mother. This daily ration of 70 g (2½ oz) of protein is guaranteed with our current nutritional recommendations. Glucose, the basic stuff of carbohydrates, is the main source of energy drawn on by the foetus. A daily intake of carbohydrates in the form of bread, pasta, or fruit is needed for a problem-free pregnancy. Fats with essential fatty acids are critical for the development and functioning of the baby's nervous system.

The increased demand for minerals and vitamins during pregnancy can be satisfied by an adequate, varied, and balanced diet. Attention should be paid to folic acid, calcium, and iron in particular, since these are often deficient.

Calcium

A substantial transfer of calcium occurs between the mother and the foetus throughout pregnancy, allowing the baby's bone and teeth formation. In the first six months, the mother stores up calcium in her own bones. When its skeletal growth reaches its peak in the last three months, the foetus draws on the mother's store. This is when the consumption of high calcium-containing foods such as milk and milk products must be increased, since a calcium deficiency will damage the mother's teeth and make her bones brittle.

Iron

The demand for iron, essential for blood formation, is also increased during pregnancy because the mother's blood volume increases, and the foetal red blood cells have to be developed. Iron is available in meat, fish, egg yolk, whole-grain products, and vegetables. Iron of plant origin is not as well assimilated as iron of animal origin. However, if you ingest vitamin C from raw food during the same meal, iron is more easily absorbed.

Folic acid

This vitamin promotes the development of the foetal central nervous system and prevents developmental defects of the neural tube (spina bifida). Folic acid is contained in vegetables, wheat germ, tropical fruits, and in eggs. However, routine nutrition does not always supply enough folic acid (vitamin B9) to meet the requirements of a pregnant woman. Additional folic acid intake is necessary in the months before pregnancy and during the first trimester.

Recommended Diet

Many factors affect the eating behavior of pregnant and lactating women; individual needs and wants, health status, social environment, selection of available foods, etc. The following recommendations ensure (in the form of a balanced diet) an adequate supply of energy, and nutritional and protective elements, and therefore represent healthy nutrition. The listed amounts and portions are averages; it is not to follow them exactly as it is in daily life.

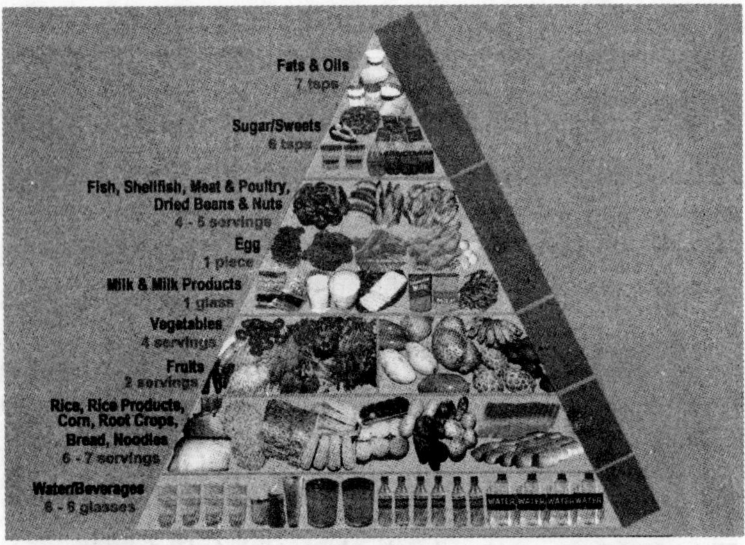
Fats & Oils
7 tsps
Sugar/Sweets
6 tsps
Fish, Shellfish, Meat & Poultry,
Dried Beans & Nuts
4 - 5 servings
Egg
1 piece
Milk & Milk Products
1 glass
Vegetables
4 servings
Fruits
2 servings
Rice, Rice Products,
Corn, Root Crops,
Bread, Noodles
6 - 7 servings
Water/Beverages
6 - 8 glasses

Fig.: Nutrition Pyramid for Lactating Women

Oils and Fats

Daily consumption: 2 teaspoons (10 g) nutritious vegetable oil such as sunflower oil, thistle oil, corn oil, unprocessed olive or canola oil, e.g., for salad dressings.

Daily consumption: at most 2 teaspoons (10 g) grease or cooking oil, such as peanut oil, or olive oil for hot meal preparation.

Daily consumption: at most 2 teaspoons (10 g) spread, i.e., butter or margarine.

Daily maximum: one meal heavy in fat such as deep fried or breaded foods, cheese dishes, fried potato cakes, bratwurst or hot dogs, cold cuts, dishes with sauces, shortcake or pastry dough, cake, pies, chocolate, etc.

Pastries/Snacks

Use them in moderation - most sweets contain hidden fat. At most eat 1 small portion of sweet snacks daily (e.g. 1 chocolate bar, 1 piece of cake or a pastry, an ice cream).

Meat, Fish, Eggs, Legumes

2-4 times per week: 1 portion meat (1 portion = 80-120 g, or 3-4 oz). More is unnecessary, less is permitted. At most, one meal of cured meats such as ham, sausage or bacon in place of meat.

At most, one meal per month of offal, such as kidney, tripe, or brains (1 portion = 80-120 g, or 3-4 oz).

Avoid Liver

1-2 portions fish per week (1 portion = 100-120 g, or 3½ -4 oz).

2-3 eggs per week, including those used in baked goods, soufflés, or cream sauces.

Properly cooked to avoid food poisoning

Per week: 1-2 portions legumes and derivates e.g., lentils, chickpeas, beans (1 portion = 40-60 g, or 1½ -2 oz, dry weight), tofu (1 portion = 100-120 g, or 3½ -4 oz)

Milk and Milk products

Per day: 3-4 portions of milk products (1 portion = 0.2 litre or ½ pint of milk, or 1 cup of yogurt, or 30 g= 1 oz hard cheese or 60 g = 2 oz soft cheese).

Grain Products and Potatoes

Daily consumption: eat 3-4 portions of starchy foods such as bread, potatoes, rice, cereals or pastas, preferably whole-grain products. The portion size depends on the frequency and amount of physical activity practiced.

Fruits

Per day: 2-3 portions of fruit, raw if at all possible (1 portion = 1 apple, 1 banana, 3 plums or a bowl of berries).

Vegetables

Per day: 2-3 portions of vegetables, one of which should be raw, e.g., as a dip vegetable or a mixed salad (1 portion = 100 g = 3½ oz raw vegetables, or 150-200 g = 5-7 oz cooked vegetables, 50 g = 1¾ oz green salad or 100 g = 3½ oz mixed salad).

Alcoholic and Non-alcoholic Drinks

Drink at least 1.5 litres (3¼ pints) of liquid per day, preferably unsweetened non-alcoholic drinks. Replace fluids in the case of vomiting, diarrhoea, or heavy perspiration.

Alcohol: for her own benefit and that of her unborn child, the pregnant mother should avoid alcohol consumption, as it is assimilated by the foetus.

By following these recommendations for correct nutrition for pregnant women, she'll ensure the health and proper development of her baby.

Nutrition for Elderly

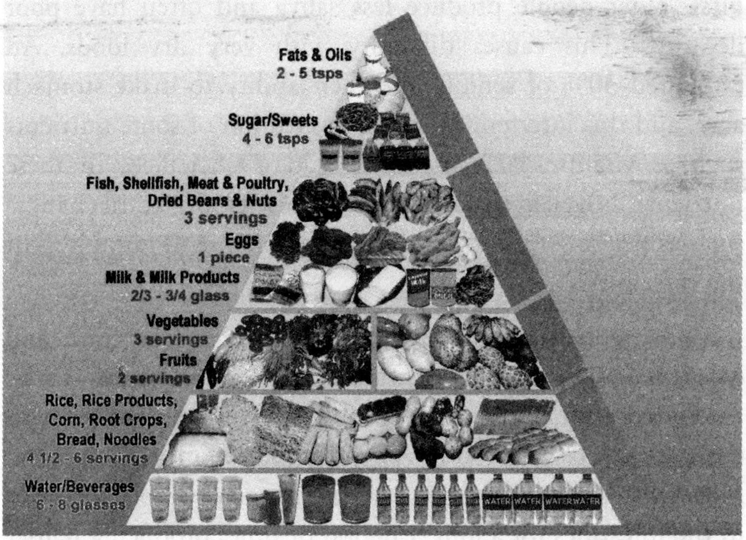

Fig.: Nutrition Pyramid for Elderly

The average life span of humans increased dramatically. Unfortunately, knowledge of the nutritional needs changes. Most nutritionists agree that nutrition is a factor in the aging process. Age-related changes in body composition and metabolism require seniors to keep a sharp eye on their food choices. Numerous elderly people are undernourished as a result of aging, eating processed and refined foods that often have lost their nutritional value, reduced metabolism, diminished appetite, and effects of medication.

Metabolic changes, along with decreased physical activity, require obtaining the same amount of nutrients from a lower caloric level. As one gets older the chances of suffering a chronic illness are greater, and health experts believe that poor eating habits contribute to some of those ailments.

Nutritional Significance of Ageing

First, older people produce less saliva and often have poor dentures. This causes difficulty with very dry foods. An estimated 30% of seniors lose their ability to make stomach acid, and this interferes with the absorption of some nutrients such as vitamin B12 and folic acid. Deficiencies in these nutrients, as well as vitamin B6, can cause neurological changes such as decline in alertness, loss of memory, and numbness of the extremities.

The reduction of the natural movement of food and enzyme activity in the gastrointestinal tract, known to be associated with aging, often results in digestive difficulties in dealing with certain foods. Also, this reduction in the natural movement of food through the intestines causes food to remain in the intestines for a longer period of time, producing harder stools and resulting in constipation. Aging affects certain senses, such as taste, smell, vision, and in tum affects the types of foods that will be chosen. Salty and sweet taste sensations can decline markedly with age, causing some to prefer foods that are richly seasoned. However, certain spicy foods produce gas. Many older persons complain of "heartburn,". that often is not caused by increased acidity but by gas production. Others resort to extra salt in order to overcome their gradual loss of taste. Sodium and its role in water retention and high blood pressure may then become a problem.

Due to certain diseases, such as heart disease or osteoporosis, elderly people need less of some minerals (such as sodium to keep lower blood pressure) and more of others (such as calcium for bone mass). Bones tend to weaken with age; evidence suggests that seniors require at least 1500 milligrams of calcium a day.

Depression and loneliness can further contribute to a disinterest in eating. Many seniors do not have the economical means, knowledge, or willingness to ensure the most nutritious choices in food selection and meal preparation, the result being malnutrition and potential health problems. Becauseof changes in the body and decreasing physical activity, older people usually need fewer calories as the rate at which the body uses energy tends to decrease. For some, food intake generally is lower, and the amount of lean body tissue decreases while the amount of body fat increases. Yet others maintain old eating habits not realizing that most people gain weight more easily as they age.

Elderly people should eat a variety of foods from five of the six major food groups (fruits; vegetables; breads and cereals; milk and cheeses; meat, poultry, fish, and dry beans) to obtain all the nutrients needed for good health. Avoid foods high in cholesterol, limit total fat intake to less than 30% of your calories and keep intake of saturated fats to less than 10%, increase your intake of dietary fibre, be selective of foods that cause gas problems, prepare moistened or softer foods,or smaller portions, if you have difficulty with dry foods. Limit the use of salt and sodium compounds, increase your calcium intake, especially elderly women, avoid too much sugar, drink at least eight (8 ounce) glasses of water daily. Alcoholic beverages should be taken in moderation. Certain drugs interact adversely with certain nutrients, so be careful about drugs. This however cannot guarantee health and well-being as health depends on many things, including heredity, lifestyle, personality traits, mental health and attitudes, and environment, in addition to one's meals.

Food alone can't make one healthy, but good eating habits based on moderation and variety can keep you healthy and even improve your health. Management of chronic health problems to improve quality of life, mobility, and independence is necessary.

Comparison of Vitamin-levels in Raw vs. Cooked Foods

The figures shown represent the amounts of vitamins per 100 grams of food, which one should keep in mind may differ from what is actually bio-available. Finally, not all cooking methods are presented here–lighter cooking methods obviously result in less vitamin losses.

Table 6: Vitamin Levels In Raw Vs. Cooked Foods
(Uncorrected for Water Loss)

Note: Amounts are expressed in units per 100g portion of food. In the table below, "boiled"=boiled, drained, without salt.

Food	Water Content (%)	Vitamin Assay				
		C (mg)	B1 (mg)	B2 (mg)	B3 (mg)	B5 (mg)
Broccoli, raw	91%	93	.065	.12	.64	.53
Broccoli, boiled	91%	75	.055	.11	.57	.51
Beef liver, raw	69%	22	.26	2.8	13	7.6
Beef liver, braised	66%	23	.20	4.1	11	4.6
Beef liver, pan-fried	56%	23	.21	4.1	14	5.9
Carrots, raw	88%	9.3	.097	.059	.93	.20
Carrots, boiled	87%	2.3	.034	.056	.51	.30
Almonds, dried	4%	.6	.21	.78	3.4	.47
Almonds, dry-roasted	3%	.7	.13	.60	2.8	.25
Mung bean sprouts, raw	90%	13	.084	.12	.75	.38
Mung bean sprouts, boiled	94%	11	.050	.10	.82	.24

Food	Water Content (%)	Vitamin Assay				
		C (mg)	B1 (mg)	B2 (mg)	B3 (mg)	B5 (mg)
Tomatoes, red, raw	94%	19	.059	.048	.63	.25
Tomatoes, boiled	92%	23	.07	.057	.75	.30
Mackerel, Atlantic, raw	63%	.4	.18	.31	9.1	.86
Mackerel, cooked, dry heat	53%	.4	.16	.41	6.8	.99
Broccoli, raw	91%	.16	71	0	1,500	1.7
Broccoli, boiled	91%	.14	50	0	1,400	1.7
Beef liver, raw	69%	.95	250	69	35,000	.67
Beef liver, braised	66%	.91	220	71	35,000	?
Beef liver, pan-fried	56%	1.4	220	112	36,000	.63
Carrots, raw	88%	.15	14	0	28,000	.46
Carrots, boiled	87%	.25	14	0	24,000	.42
Almonds, dried	4%	.11	59	0	0	24
Almonds, dry-roasted	3%	.07	64	0	0	5.5
Mung bean sprouts, raw	90%	.09	61	0	21	.01

Food	Water Content (%)	Vitamin Assay				
		C (mg)	B1 (mg)	B2 (mg)	B3 (mg)	B5 (mg)
Mung bean sprouts, boiled	94%	.05	29	0	14	.01
Tomatoes, red, raw	94%	.08	15	0	620	.38
Tomatoes, boiled	92%	.09	13	0	740	.38
Mackerel, Atlantic, raw	63%	.40	1.3	8.7	165	1.5
Mackerel, cooked, dry heat	53%	.46	1.5	19	180	?

Here is the Average Vitamin Loss, expressed in Percentages, and Corrected for the Effect of Water Loss

Table 7: Vitamin Losses From Cooking
(Corrected for Water Loss)
Expressed as Average Percentage Decrease from Value Observed in Raw Food.

Food	Water Content	Vitamin Assay				
		C	B1	B2	B3	B5
Average Losses (% lost compared to Raw value)						
Uncorrected for water loss	8	8	18	-11	10	9
Corrected for water loss	--	16	26	-3	18	17
Food	**Water Content**	**Vitamin Assay**				
		B6	**Folate**	**B12**	**A**	**E**
Average Losses (% lost compared to Raw value)						
Uncorrected for water loss	8	-5	12	?	3	3
Corrected for water loss	--	3	20	?	11	11

Table 8: Mineral Levels In Raw Vs. Cooked Foods

(Uncorrected for Water Loss)

Note: Amounts are expressed in Units per 100g portion of Food. In the table below, "boiled"= boiled, drained, without salt.

Food	Water Content	Mineral Assay (all amounts in mg)								
		Ca	Fe	Mg	P	K	Na	Zn	Cu	Mn
Broccoli, raw	91%	48	.88	25	66	320	27	.40	.045	.23
Broccoli, boiled	91%	46	.84	24	59	290	26	.38	.043	.22
Beef liver, raw	69%	6	6.8	19	320	320	73	3.9	3.3	.26
Beef liver, braised	66%	7	6.8	20	400	230	70	6.1	4.5	.41
Beef liver, pan-fried	56%	11	6.3	23	460	360	110	5.4	4.5	.42
Carrots, raw	88%	27	.50	15	44	320	35	.20	.047	.14
Carrots, boiled	87%	31	.62	13	30	230	66	.30	.13	.75
Almonds, dried	4%	270	3.7	290	520	730	11	2.9	.94	2.3
Almonds, dry roasted	3%	280	3.8	300	550	770	11	4.9	1.2	2.0
Mung bean sprouts, raw	90%	13	.91	21	54	150	6	.41	.16	.19
Mung bean sprouts, boiled	94%	12	.65	14	28	101	10	.47	.12	.14

Food	Water Content	Mineral Assay (all amounts in mg)								
		Ca	Fe	Mg	P	K	Na	Zn	Cu	Mn
Tomatoes, red, raw	94%	5	.45	11	24	220	6	.09	.074	.10
Tomatoes, boiled	92%	6	.56	14	31	280	11	.11	.093	.13
Mackerel, Atlantic, raw	63%	12	1.6	76	220	310	90	.63	.073	.01
Mackerel, cooked, dry heat	53%	15	1.6	97	280	400	83	.94	.090	.02

Balanced Diets

Balanced Diets For Adult Men*

Dietary Articles	Sedentary Work		Moderate Work		Heavy Work	
	Vegetarian (gm)	Non-vegetarian (gm)	Vegetarian (gm)	Non-vegetarian (gm)	Vegetarian (gm)	Non-vegetarian (gm)
Cereals	400	400	475	475	650	650
Pulses	70	55	80	65	80	65
Green Leafy Vegetables	100	100	125	125	125	125
Other Vegetables	75	75	75	75	100	100
Roots and Tubers	75	75	100	100	100	100
Fruits	30	30	30	30	30	30
Milk	300	100	300	100	300	100
Fats and Oils	40	35	45	40	50	45
Meat and Fish	–	30	–	50	–	60
Egg	–	30	–	30	–	30
Sugar and Jaggery	30	30	40	40	55	55
Groundnuts	–	–	–	–	50	50

Balanced Diets For Adult Women*

Dietary Articles	Sedentary Work		Moderate Work		Heavy Work		Additional Allowance During	
	Vegetarian (gm)	Non-vegetarian (gm)	Vegetarian (gm)	Non-vegetarian (gm)	Vegetarian (gm)	Non-vegetarian (gm)	Pregnancy (gm)	Lactation (gm)
Cereals	300	300	350	350	475	475	50	100
Pulses	60	45	70	55	70	55	–	10
Green Leafy Vegetables	125	125	125	125	125	125	25	25
Other Vegetables	75	75	75	75	10	100	–	–
Roots and Tubers	50	50	75	75	100	100	–	–
Fruits	30	30	30	30	30	30	–	–
Milk	200	100	200	100	200	100	125	125
Fats and Oils	35	30	40	35	50	45	–	15
Meat and Fish	–	30	–	30	–	50	–	–
Egg	–	30	–	40	–	30	–	–
Sugar and Jaggery	30	30	30	30	40	40	10	20
Groundnuts	–	–	–	–	40	40	–	–

Balance Diets For Adult Children*

Dietary Articles	Pre-school Children				School Children			
	1-3 years		4-6 years		7-9 years		10-12 years	
	Vegetarian (gm)	Non-vegetarian (gm)	Vegetarian (gm)	Non-vegetarian (gm)	Vegetarian (gm)	Non-vegetarian (gm)	Vegetarian (gm)	Non-vegetarian (gm)
Cereals	150	150	200	200	250	250	320	310
Pulses	50	40	60	50	70	60	70	60
Green Leafy Vegetables	50	50	75	75	75	75	100	100
Other Vegetables	30	30	50	50	50	50	75	75
Roots and Tubers	50	50	50	50	60	60	60	60
Fruits	500	200	400	200	500	200	400	200
Milk	20	25	25	25	30	30	35	35
Fats and Oils	–	30	–	30	40	40	–	50
Meat and Fish	30	30	40	40	50	50	50	50
Egg	30	30	40	40	50	50	50	50
Sugar and Jaggery	30	30	40	40	50	50	50	50

Balanced Diets For Adolescent Boys And Girls*

Dietary Articles	Boys				Girls	
	13-15 years		16-18 years		13-18 years	
	Vegetarian (gm)	Non-vegetarian (gm)	Vegetarian (gm)	Non-vegetarian (gm)	Vegetarian (gm)	Non-vegetarian (gm)
Cereals	430	430	450	450	350	350
Pulses	70	50	70	50	70	50
Green Leafy Vegetables	100	100	100	100	150	150
Other Vegetables	75	75	75	75	75	75
Roots and Tubers	75	75	100	100	75	75
Fruits	30	30	30	30	30	30
Milk	500	200	400	150	400	150
Fats and Oils	35	40	45	50	35	40
Meat and Fish	–	60	–	70	–	80
Egg	–	30	–	30	–	30
Sugar and Jaggery	30	30	40	40	30	30
Groundnuts	–	–	50	50	–	–

*Adapted from tables on Balanced Diets as given in the report of the Nutrition Expert Group, Indian Council of Medical Research, New Delhi.

Chart Showing Average Iron Contents In Some Vegetables, Fruits & Animal Products

In mg. per 100 gm.	
Banana (Unripe)	0.6
Banana Plant (Stem)	1.1
Fruits-buds of Banana Plant	1.6
Fig	1.0
Apple	1.0
Spinach	10.9
Mustard Leaves	16.3
Buckwheat Leaves	16.5
Coriander Leaves	18.5
Gram Leaves	23.8
Margosa Leaves (Young)	25.3
Arum Leave-stalks (Brown Variety)	38.7
Cauliflower (with Leaves)	40.0
Egg (Hen)	2.1
Egg (Duck)	3.0
Liver	6.3

Chart Showing Average Vitamin A Contents In Some Vegetables

In International Units Per 100 gm.	
Mustard Leaves	1300.00
Carrot	1800.00
Buckwheat Leaves	2300.00
Spinach	5600.00
Horse-raddish Leaves	7000.00

9
Ideal Diet Plan

Proper diet with exercises help you stay healthy.

For Pure Vegans

A 1,200-calorie eating plan designed to help you stay slim trim and satisfied. This diet is split in 4 weeks period with the diet changing every week.

d. Before starting the diet weigh yourself and write it down somewhere. This way you know w here you started and you feel good to see the scales going down.

Some things you need to follow this diet: No salt after 7:30PM.

No aerated drinks. Yes that includes even the diet version. Restrict mango and banana.

Restrict potato and rice.

No artificial juices as well.

Half an hour of aerobic exercise daily. If you want to join a gym good enough. But if due to any reason maybe time or money constraint you can't join a gym. All you need is a comfortable pair of shoes to do some aerobics, a skipping rope to do at least 500 skips (5 sets of 100 skips and increasing it as you go). 1.5 -2 kgs dumbbells for toning your upper body. Just these basic things and you are set.

20 mins of breathing exercise. (*pranayam*)

Now I present you with the Indian diet plan:

Week 1

8:00 am (as soon as you wake up) – 2 glasses of methi seeds water (soak 1 tsp of methi seeds in 2 glasses of water. Strain out the methi seeds and drink the water. Helps a lot in water retention and bloating) 5 soaked almonds with the skin. 1 kali mirch you don't have to chew it just swallow it down.

9:00 am – 1 toast (brown bread) with amul lite butter / hung curd dressing/ salad and chutney

11:30 am – one fruit of your wish

1:30 pm – A small plate of salad before starting the meal. The fibres in the salad fills you up which in turn prevents false hunger that makes you overeat.1 bran chappati (mix wheat flour and wheat bran in equal proportions.) with 1 bowl (normal sized katori) of dal. Generally at my place dal is cooked at night so I used to store the dal made at night for the other days lunch, you can do the same.

5:00 pm – 1cup of milk or tea with 2 biscuits(just marie, no other biscuits)/ 1 small bowl bhuna channa/ 1bowl popcorn (not the buttery act 2 ones but air popped popcorns without the butter)

7:30 pm –A small plate of salad before starting the meal. 1 bran chappati with 1 k vegetable (any vegetable not rajmah, channa or kadhi)

8:30 pm – one fruit of your wish

When this week ends, weigh yourself again. I'm sure u must have lost weight. I lost 1.8kgs in the first week itself. U lose the max in this week because you lose all the water weight and the bloating is gone. The further weeks you are surely going to lose weight but it won't be this much.

Week 2

8:00 am (as soon as you wake up) – 2 glasses of tulsi leave water (soak 5 tulsi leaves in 2 glasses of water. Strain out the leaves and drink the water.) 5 soaked almonds with the skin. 1 kali mirch.

9:00 am – 1 toast (brown bread) with amul lite butter/ hung curd dressing/salad and chutney

11:30 am – one fruit of your wish

1:30 pm – A small plate of salad before starting the meal. 1 sandwich (2 brown breads with paneer filling, if you are a vegetarian and egg whites, if you are a non vegetarian.)

5:00 pm – 1cup of milk or tea with 2 biscuits

7:30 pm –A small plate of salad before starting the meal. 1 bran chappati with 1 k vegetable (this week you can take rajma, channa or kadhi)

8:30 pm – one fruit of your wish

This week I lost just 9 kgs

Week 3

8:00 am – 2 glasses of methi seeds water. 5 soaked almonds with the skin. 1 kali mirch.

9:00 am - 1 glass of milk and a fruit

11:30 am – one fruit of your wish

1:30 pm – 1 bran chappati and any vegetable

5:00 pm – 1cup of milk or tea with 2 biscuits/1 small bowl bhuna channa/1bowl popcorn (not the buttery act 2 ones but air popped popcorns without the butter)

7:30 pm – 3 pcs steamed or roasted chicken or fish + salad (non vegetarians)

Any one of the following for vegetarians:

1. 1 bowl dal + 1 bowl curd + salad
2. 1 bowl veg + 1 bowl curd + salad

8:30 pm – one fruit of your wish

Week 4

8:00 am - 2 glasses of methi seeds water. 5 soaked almonds with the skin. 1 kali mirch.

9:00 am - 1 glass of cold coffee and a bread butter toast

11:30 am – one fruit of your wish

1:30 pm – This week you have a lot of options which you can take alternatively.

1 bowl sprouts + fruits

2 bowl vegetables + salads

1 bowl dalia + 1 bb toast

1 bowl vegetables + 1 bb toast

1 bowl kadhi + 1 quarter plate rice

5:00 pm - 1cup of milk or tea with 2 biscuits/ 1 small bowl bhuna channa/1 bowl popcorn (not the buttery act 2 ones but air popped popcorns without the butter)

7:30 pm – 1 bran chappati and 1 bowl vegetable.

8:30 pm – one fruit of your wish

Don't let suffer your social life while on a diet plan, you can still manage your weight without locking yourself at home. Some pointers for it:

When you go out with friends try to have your lunch or dinner at subway. The healthiest option out there. Take a veggie delite sub in brown bread and eating out won't harm your diet and weight at all. Tell them not to put mayo in it though.

If you don't have a say in the place of eating then make your choices sensibly. If you go to eat Chinese have rice rather than noodles. Order stir fried veggies instead of Manchurian. And control your proportions. Don't take fried starters. Avoid those thick soups they are no good.

When going out just pick 2 fruits before sitting in the car and eat it on your way to the venue. When you are already a little filled before going out. Your somewhat filled stomach helps your mind take the right decision.

If eating Indian, order tandoori chappati rather than butter naan or parantha. Take less gravy since it is the most fattening.

Keep these points in your mind and you will be able to maintain your weight easily.

Bengali Diet Program

Summerizing the bengali cuisine in 1200 calories was the most difficult task. Being born and raised as a Bengali may make you experience the pleasures hidden in the water! In other words, your Bengali soul and spirit may get enriched with the pleasures that you derive from the great taste of fish recipes. Bengalis and East Indians in general, are known for their love of fish dishes! In fact, the Bengali recipes have earned a worldwide recognition.

When we talk about Bengalis, we'll certainly discuss about "Machher Jhol', "Rui Machher Kalia", Bhetki Fry and "Ilisher

Paturi"! As you know, oil and spice concentrations are the major building blocks of a great taste, so it means that you are not taking in loads of calories from the oil alone, but the incredible taste is also urging you to eat more and more. Under such a situation, you may not know when and how to put a "full stop". But your doctor, neighbors and other well-wishers have also asked you to keep a check on your weight! You may find a sample 1200 Calorie Bengali Diet Plan for Weight Loss working for you:

Bengali Diet Plan for Weight Loss (1200 Calorie)

Food Item	Amount	Calories (KCal)	Protein (gms.)
Breakfast (8:00- 9:00 am)			
Rice Cheela with Onions	2	200	3
Or, Besan Cheela with Onions	2	200	12
Tea/Coffee (with 50ml. Milk)	150ml.	125	2
Apple	1	30	-
Mid-Morning (11:00 – 12:00 noon)			
Buttermilk 150ml.	-	20	1
Or, Sprouts Salad	100gms.	100	6
Lunch (1:00 – 2:00 pm)			
Wheat Bran Chapati (No Oil)	2	200	6
Chicken Curry	50gms.	200	8
Or, Arhar Dal	50gms.	150	6
Salad	100gms.	40	1
Evening (4:00 – 5:00 pm)			
Murmura Chaat	100gms.	40	2
Or, Steamed Corn	100gms.	40	-
Tea/Coffee (with 50ml. Milk)	150 ml	125	2

Food Item	Amount	Calories (KCal)	Protein (gms.)
Dinner (8:00 – 9:00p m)			
Poha with Onions and Tomato	100gms.	150	2
Or, Wheat Bran Chapati	1	100	3
Green Veg. Salad	100gms.	40	1
Total (approximately)		**1200**	**40**

It is admitted that our "provoked" tongue will always try to lick the hot and spicy fishes and then again, it will attempt to venture with the other extreme taste- the taste of Mitha Dahi, Rasgullas, Amriti, Chhanar Pulav, Sheeta Bhog, Chitrakoot and Khejur Gurer Payesh. This is the Bengali tradition – ending up a meal with some heart-warming sweet dishes! The fact is that, you can enjoy all the goodness in the East Indian cuisine and keep a control on the calorie meter provided you check your portion intakes. Remember, all the good things come in small packets!

An Ideal Bengali Diet Plan

An Ideal Bengali diet plan can be designed keeping in mind the person's individual requirements. Every person has different caloric requirement. the calorie requirement is based on various factors like age, sex, medical conditions, activity levels, metabolism etc. To Lose weight in a healthy manner, calculate your BMR (Basal Metabolic Rate). This will help you in knowing how many minimum calories your body requires in order to function properly.

This Sample Bengali diet plan will provide you with an idea of what ideally a 1200 calorie Bengali meal looks like. Although you must understand that this is just a generalized Bengali diet plan for weight loss, it may or may not suit your weight loss goal as there are chances your body requirements will be different. So do consult your dietician in person to know if you can use this 1200 calorie Bengali Diet plan for weight loss.

For Non Vegans

A 1,500-calorie eating Non Veg plan designed to help you stay trim and satisfied.

Breakfast

2 egg stuffed omelette (mushroom and onion), 1 slice of multi-grain toast with a slice of low- fat cheese, 1 cup of black coffee (add milk and stevia, if desired). According to the US National Institute of Health, people who have a high-protein breakfast are more likely to feel full throughout the day than those who consume protein any another time.

Snack

1 cup fresh yoghurt (whipped) 1/2 cup fresh strawberries, halved 1 apple, chopped 1 tsp flaxseed 6 almonds and 5 walnuts *Studies show that the longer you chew on almonds, the more you may absorb their healthy, satiety-boosting fats. Total: 220 calories.

Lunch

Chicken salad with vinaigrette: 150 g roast chicken pieces (you can also use smoked chicken) 6-8 pieces sun-dried tomatoes 1 apple, chopped 30 g olives vinaigrette to taste 3-4 Tbsp of olive oil 1 cup mixed greens (lettuce, spinach, rocket leaves), 1 slice of multi-grain toast. Lean protein such as chicken is vital when you cut calories because it fills you up without a lot of fat and helps you build muscle too. Total: 450 calories

Snack

1 cup moong bean sprouts 15 peanuts Salt, pepper and lemon to taste A small mocha latte from your nearest coffee shop (174 Kcals) Total: 290 calories

Dinner

Steamed fish fillets with grilled garden vegetables, 1 cup of home-made tomato soup 200 g steamed or grilled fish, 1 cup grilled vegetables. According to the International Society for the Study of Fatty Acids and Lipids, the Omega-3 in tuna helps reduce the risk of becoming obese and improve the body's ability to respond to insulin. Total: 250 calories

Daily total:

1,500 calories

Note: For optimal weight management, combine this nutrient-dense meal plan with exercise at least 4-5 times a week.

Dinner

Steamed fish fillets with grilled garden vegetables. 1 cup of home-made tomato soup, 200 g steamed or grilled fish, 1 cup grilled vegetables. According to the International Society for the Study of Fatty Acids and Lipids, the Omega-3 in tuna helps reduce the risk of becoming obese and improve the body's ability to respond to insulin. Total: 250 calories.

Daily total

1,500 calories

Note: For optimal weight management, combine this nutrient-dense meal plan with exercise at least 4–5 times a week.

10
The Food Pyramid

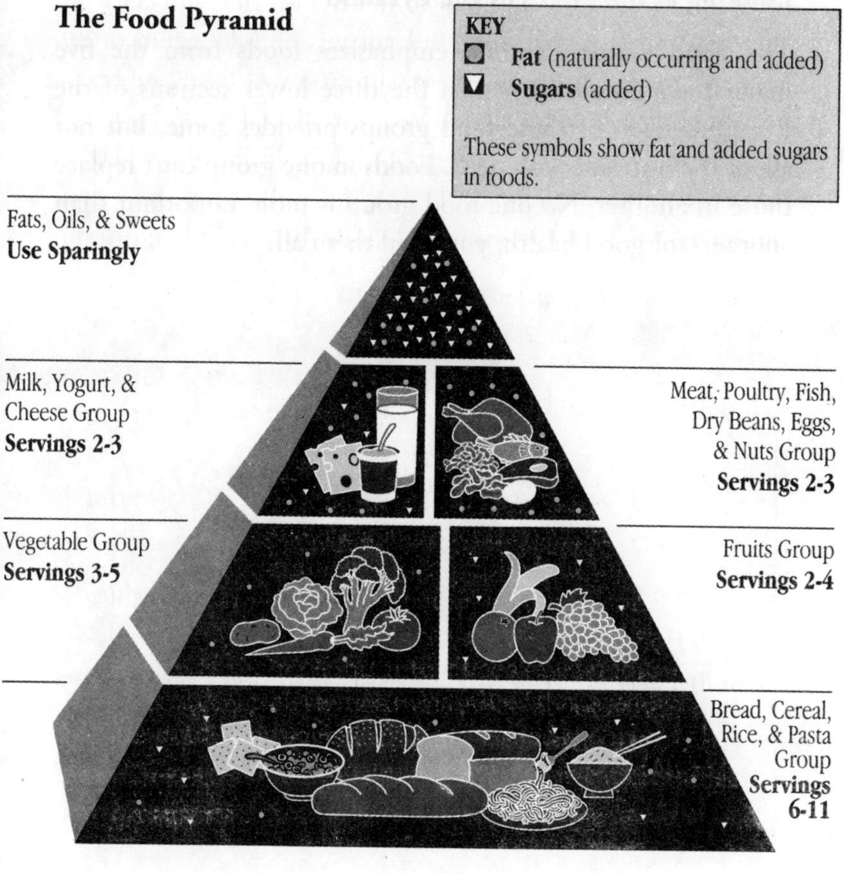

What is the Food Guide Pyramid?

The Pyramid is an outline of what to eat each day. It's not a rigid prescription, but a general guide that lets you choose a healthful diet that's right for you.

The Pyramid calls for eating a variety of foods to get the nutrients you need and at the same time the right amount of calories to maintain or improve your weight.

The Pyramid also focuses on fat because most people diets are too high in fat, especially saturated fat.

Looking at the Pieces of the Pyramid

The Food Guide Pyramid emphasizes foods from the five major food groups shown in the three lower sections of the Pyramid. Each of these food groups provides some, but not all, of the nutrients you need. Foods in one group can't replace those in another. No one food group is more important than another–for good health, you need them all.

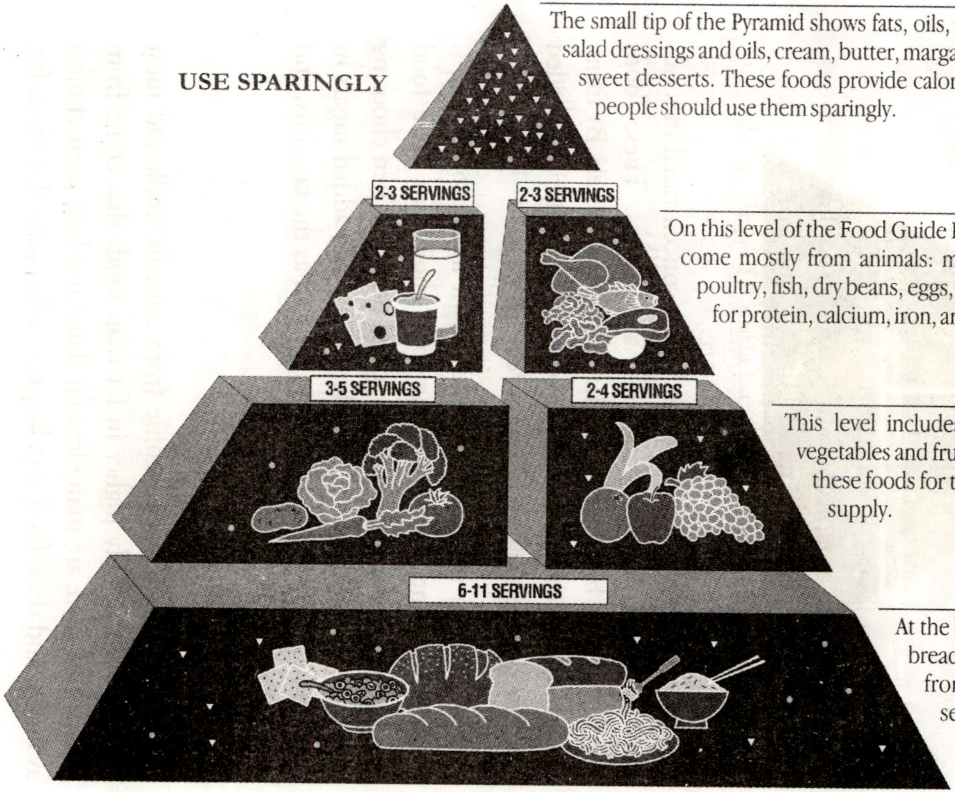

The small tip of the Pyramid shows fats, oils, and sweets. These are foods such as salad dressings and oils, cream, butter, margarine, sugars, soft drinks, candies, and sweet desserts. These foods provide calories and little else nutritionally. Most people should use them sparingly.

On this level of the Food Guide Pyramid are two groups of foods that come mostly from animals: milk, yogurt, and cheese; and meat, poultry, fish, dry beans, eggs, and nuts. These foods are important for protein, calcium, iron, and zinc.

This level includes foods that come from plants – vegetables and fruits. Most people need to eat more of these foods for the vitamins, minerals, and fibre they supply.

At the base of the Food Guide Pyramid are breads, cereals, rice, and pasta—all foods from grains. You need the most servings of these foods each day.

A Closer Look at Fat and Added Sugars

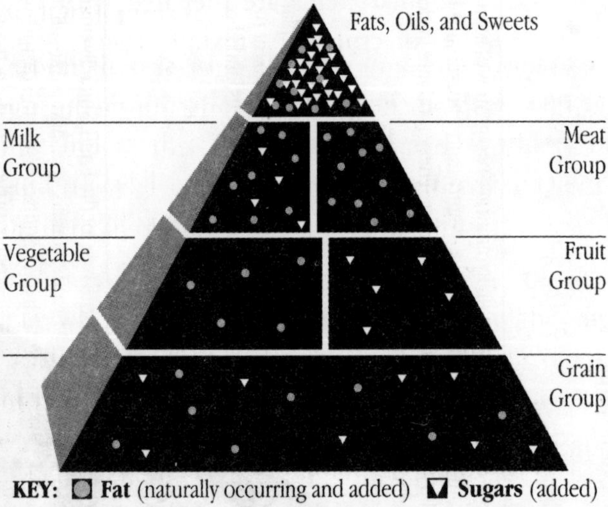

As you can see, fat and added sugars are concentrated in foods from the Pyramid tip—fats, oils, and sweets. These foods supply calories, but little or no vitamins and minerals. By using these foods sparingly, you can have a diet that supplies needed vitamins and minerals without excess calories.

Some fat or sugar symbols are shown in the food groups. That's to remind you that some food choices in these food groups can also be high in fat or added sugars. When choosing foods for a healthful diet, consider the fat and added sugars in your choices from the food groups, as well as the fats, oils, and sweets from the Pyramid tip.

Fat

In general, foods that come from animals (milk and meat groups) are naturally higher in fat than foods that come from plants. But there are many low-fat dairy and lean meat choices available, and these foods can be prepared in ways that lower fat.

Fruits, vegetables, and grain products are naturally low in fat. But many popular items are prepared with fat, like french-fried potatoes or croissants, making them higher fat choices.

For example:

One Baked Potato		**14 French Fries**
Calories: 120		Calories: 225
Fat: trace	*Or*	Fat: 11 grams

Added Sugars

▼ These symbols represent sugars added to foods in processing or at the table, not the sugars found naturally in fruits and milk. It's the added sugars that provide calories with few vitamins and minerals.

Most of the added sugars in the typical American diet come from foods in the Pyramid tip—soft drinks, candy, jams, jellies, syrups, and table sugar we add to foods like coffee or cereal.

Added sugars in the food groups come from foods such as ice cream, sweetened yogurt, chocolate milk, canned or frozen fruit with heavy syrup, and sweetened bakery products like cakes and cookies. The table on pages 152-53 shows you the amounts of added sugars in some popular foods. You may be surprised!

Fat and Sugar Tips

☞ Choose lower fat foods from the food groups most often.

☞ Go easy on fats and sugars added to foods in cooking or at the table—butter, margarine, gravy, salad dressing, sugar, and jelly.

☞ Choose fewer foods that are high in sugars—candy, sweet desserts, and soft drinks.

How To Make the Pyramid Work for You

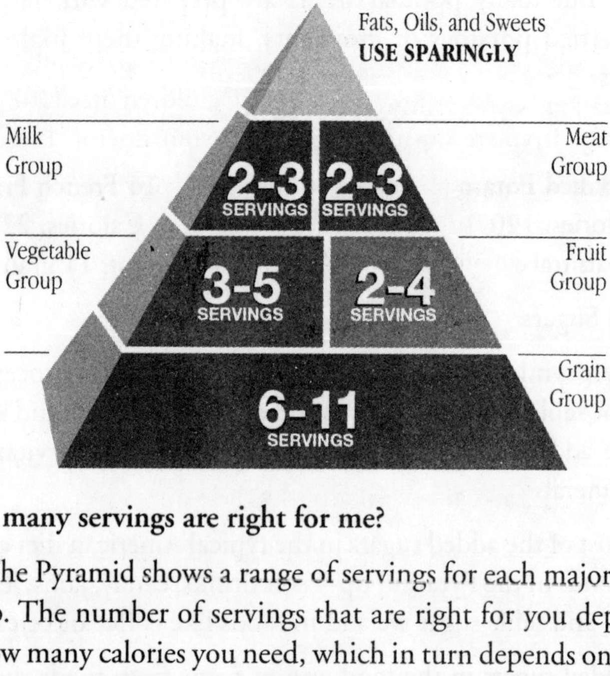

How many servings are right for me?

The Pyramid shows a range of servings for each major food group. The number of servings that are right for you depends on how many calories you need, which in turn depends on your age, sex, size, and how active you are. Almost everyone should have at least the lowest number of servings in the ranges.

The following calorie level suggestions are based on recommendations of the National Academy of Sciences and on calorie intakes reported by people in national food consumption surveys.

For adults and teens

1,600 calories is about right for many sedentary women and some older adults.

2,200 calories is about right for most children, teenage girls, active women, and many sedentary men. Women who are pregnant or breastfeeding may need somewhat more.

2,800 calories is about right for teenage boys, many active men, and some very active women.

For young children

It is hard to know how much food children need to grow normally. If you're unsure, check with your doctor. Preschool children need the same variety of foods as older family members do, but may need less than 1,600 calories. For fewer calories they can eat smaller servings. However, it is important that they have the equivalent of 2 cups of milk a day.

For you

Now, take a look at the table below. It tells you how many servings you need for your calorie level. For example, if you are an active woman who needs about 2,200 calories a day, 9 servings of breads, cereals, rice, or pasta would be right for you. You'd also want to eat about 6 ounces of meat or alternates per day. Keep total fat (fat in the foods you choose as well as fat used in cooking or added at the table) to about 73 grams per day.

If you are between calorie categories, estimate servings. For example, some less active women may need only 2,000 calories to maintain a healthy weight. At that calorie level, 8 servings of breads would be about right.

Sample Diets For A Day At 3 Calorie Levels

	Lower about 1,600	Moderate about 2,200	Higher about 2,800
Grain Group Servings	6	9	11
Vegetable Group Servings	3	4	5
Fruit Group Servings	2	3	4

	Lower about 1,600	Moderate about 2,200	Higher about 2,800
Milk Group Servings	2-3[1]	2-3[1]	2-3[1]
Meat Group[2] (ounces)	5	6	7
Total Fat[3] (grams)	53	73	93
Total Added Sugars[4] (teaspoons)	6	12	18

1 Women who are pregnant or breastfeeding, teenagers, and young adults to age 24 need 3 servings.

2 Meat group amounts are in total ounces.

3 See the Pyramid Food Choices Chart for details on how to count total fat.

4 How to count teaspoons of added sugars has been discussed above.

What is a Serving?

The amount of food that counts as a serving is listed on the next page. If you eat a larger portion, count it as more than one serving. For example, 1/2 cup of cooked pasta counts as one serving in the bread, cereal, rice, and pasta group. If you eat 1 cup of pasta, that would be two servings. If you eat a smaller portion, count it as part of a serving.

Isn't 6 to 11 servings of breads and cereals a lot?

It may sound like a lot, but it's really not. For example, a slice of bread is one serving, so a sandwich for lunch would equal two servings. A small bowl of cereal and one slice of toast for breakfast are two more servings. And, if you have a cup of rice or pasta at dinner, that's two more servings. A snack of 3 or 4 small plain crackers adds yet another serving. So now you've had 7 servings. It adds up quicker than you think!

Do I need to measure servings?

No. Use servings only as a general guide. For mixed foods, do the best you can to estimate the food group servings of the main ingredients. For example, a generous serving of pizza would count in the grain group (crust), the milk group (cheese), and the vegetable group (tomato); a helping of beef stew would count in the meat group and the vegetable group. Both have some fat — fat in the cheese on the pizza and in the gravy from the stew, if it's made from meat drippings.

What if I want to lose or gain weight?

The best and simplest way to lose weight is to increase your physical activity and reduce the fat and sugars in your diet. But be sure to eat at least the lowest number of servings from the five major food groups in the Food Guide Pyramid. You need them for the vitamins, minerals, carbohydrates, and protein they provide. Just try to pick the lowest fat choices from the food groups.

To gain weight, increase the amounts of foods you eat from all of the food groups. If you have lost weight unexpectedly, see your doctor.

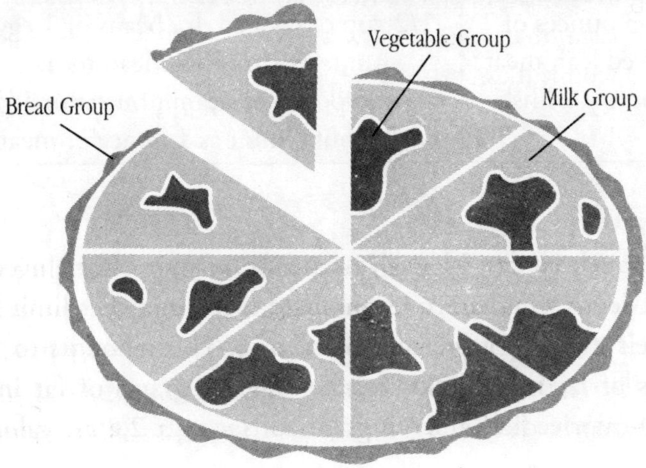

What Counts As A Serving?

Food Groups

Bread, Cereal, Rice, and Pasta		
1 slice of bread	1 ounce of ready-to-eat cereal	1/2 cup of cooked cereal, rice, or pasta
Vegetable		
1 cup of raw leafy vegetables	1/2 cup of other vegetables, cooked or chopped raw	3/4 cup of vegetable juice
Fruit		
1 medium apple, banana, orange	1/2 cup of chopped, cooked, or canned fruit	3/4 cup of fruit juice
Milk, Yogurt, and Cheese		
1 cup of milk or yogurt	1-1/2 ounces of natural cheese	2 ounces of process cheese
Meat, Poultry, Fish, Dry Beans, Eggs and Nuts		
2-3 ounces of cooked lean meat, poultry, or fish	1/2 cup of cooked dry beans or 1 egg counts as 1 ounce of lean meat. 2 tablespoons of peanut butter or 1/3 cup of nuts count as 1 ounce of meat.	

Fats

How much fat can I have? It depends on your calorie needs. The Dietary Guidelines recommend that Americans limit fat in their diets to 30 percent of calories. This amounts to 53 grams of fat in a 1,600- calorie diet, 73 grams of fat in a 2,200-calorie diet, and 93 grams of fat in a 2,800- calorie diet.

You will get up to half this fat even if you pick the lowest fat choices from each food group and add no fat to your foods in preparation or at the table.

You decide how to use the additional fat in your daily diet. You may want to have foods from the five major food groups that are higher in fat such as whole milk instead of skim milk. Or you may want to use it in cooking or at the table in the form of spreads, dressings, or toppings.

How to check your diet for fat

If you want to be sure you have a low fat diet, you can count the grams of fat in your day's food choices using the Pyramid Food Choices Chart, and compare them to the number of grams of fat suggested for your calorie level.

You don't need to count fat grams every day, but doing a fat check-up once in awhile will help keep you on the right track. If you find you are eating too much fat, choose lower fat foods more often.

Are some types of fat worse than others?

Yes. Eating too much saturated fat raises blood cholesterol levels in many people, increasing their risk for heart disease. The Dietary Guidelines recommend limiting saturated fat to less than 10 percent of calories, or about one-third of total fat intake.

All fats in foods are mixtures of three types of fatty acids—saturated, monounsaturated, and polyunsaturated.

Saturated fats are found in largest amounts in fats from meat and dairy products and in some vegetable fats such as coconut, palm, and palm kernel oils.

Monounsaturated fats are found mainly in olive, peanut, and canola oils.

Polyunsaturated fats are found mainly in safflower, sunflower, corn, soybean, and cottonseed oils and some fish.

You can figure the number of grams of fat that provide **30%** of calories in your daily diet as follows:

A. Multiply your total day's calories by 0.30 to get your calories from fat per day. Example: 2,200 calories x 0.30 = 660 calories from fat.

B. Divide calories from fat per day by 9 (each gram of fat has 9 calories) to get grams of fat per day. Example: 660 calories from fat ÷ 9 = 73 grams of fat

Where's The Fat?

Bologna	= 16 grams
Cheese	= 12 grams
Mayonnaise	= 8 grams
	36 grams or 9 teaspoons of fat

The fat in some foods adds up quickly. A bologna-and-cheese sandwich made with 2 slices (2 oz.) of bologna, 2 slices (1-1/2 oz.) of cheese, and 2 teaspoons of mayonnaise counts up to about 36 grams of fat, about 9 teaspoons. However, a similar sandwich made with lean beef, lettuce, tomato, and low-fat mayonnaise, and served with a cup of non-fat milk instead of the cheese, has only about 6 grams of fat.

Note: 4 grams of fat = 1 teaspoon

How do I avoid too much saturated fat?

Follow the Food Guide Pyramid, keeping your total fat within recommended levels. Choose fat from a variety of food sources, but mostly from those foods that are higher in polyunsaturated or monounsaturated fat.

Here are some selection tips:

- ☞ Use lean meats and skim or low-fat dairy products.
- ☞ Use unsaturated vegetable oils and margarines that list a liquid vegetable oil as first ingredient on the label.
- ☞ Read nutrition and ingredient labels on food packages to check the kinds and amounts of fat they contain.
- ☞ Limit use of products that contain a large amount of saturated fats. Examples are non-dairy creamers and rich baked products such as pie crusts and other pastries, cakes, and cookies.

Cholesterol

What about cholesterol?

Cholesterol and fat are not the same thing. Cholesterol is a fat-like substance present in all animal foods—meat, poultry, fish, milk and milk products, and egg yolks. Both the lean and fat of meat and the meat and skin of poultry contain cholesterol. In milk products, cholesterol is mostly in the fat, so lower fat products contain less cholesterol. Egg yolks and organ meats, like liver, are high in cholesterol. Plant foods do not contain cholesterol.

Dietary cholesterol, as well as saturated fat, raises blood cholesterol levels in many people, increasing their risk for heart disease. Some health authorities recommend that dietary cholesterol be limited to an average of 300 mg or less per day. To keep dietary cholesterol to this level, follow the Food Guide Pyramid, keeping your total fat to the amount that's right for you. (See table on pages 145-46.) It's not necessary to eliminate all foods that are high in cholesterol. You can have three to four egg yolks a week, counting those used as ingredients in custards and baked products. Use lower fat dairy products often and occasionally include dry beans and peas in place of meat.

Where's The Cholesterol?

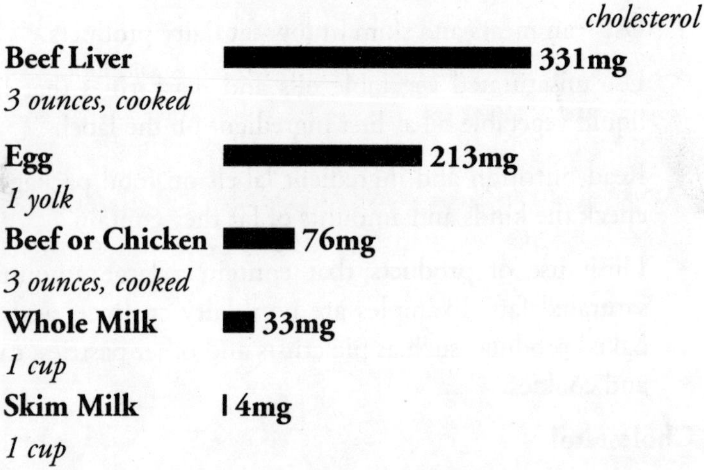

Where Are The Added Sugars?

Food Groups	Added Sugars (teaspoons)
Bread, Cereal, Rice, and Pasta	
Bread, 1 slice	0
Muffin, 1 medium	★1
Cookies, 2 medium	★1
Danish pastry, 1 medium	★1
Doughnut, 1 medium	★★2
Ready-to-eat cereal, sweetened, 1 oz.	*
Pound cake, no-fat, 1 oz.	★★2
Angelfood cake, 1/12 tube cake	★★★★★5
Cake, frosted, 1/16 average	★★★★★★6
Pie, fruit, 2 crust, 1/6 8" pie	★★★★★★6
Fruit	
Fruit, canned in juice, 1/2 cup	0

Food Groups	Added Sugars (teaspoons)
Fruit, canned in light syrup, 1/2 cup	★★2
Fruit, canned in heavy syrup, 1/2 cup	★★★★4
Milk, Yogurt, and Cheese	
Milk, plain, 1 cup	0
Chocolate milk, 2 percent, 1 cup	★★★3
Low-fat yogurt, plain, 8 oz.	0
Low-fat yogurt, flavoured, 8 oz.	★★★★★5
Low-fat yogurt, fruit, 8 oz.	★★★★★★★7
Ice cream, ice milk, or frozen yogurt, 1/2 cup	★★★3
Chocolate shake, 10 fl. oz.	★★★★★★★★★9
Other	
Sugar, jam, or jelly, 1 tsp.	★1
Syrup or honey, 1 tbsp.	★★★3
Chocolate bar, 1 oz.	★★★3
Fruit sorbet, 1/2 cup	★★★3
Gelatin dessert, 1/2 cup	★★★★4
Sherbet, 1/2 cup	★★★★★5
Cola, 12 fl.oz.	★★★★★★★★★9
Fruit drink, ade, 12 fl.oz.	★★★★★★★★★★★★12

*Check product label ★ = 1 teaspoon sugar

Note: 4 grams of sugar = 1 teaspoon

Sugars

What about sugars?

Choosing a diet low in fat is a concern for everyone; choosing one low in sugars is also important for people who have low calorie needs. Sugars include white sugar, brown sugar, raw sugar, corn syrup, honey, and molasses; these supply calories and little else nutritionally.

To avoid getting too many calories from sugars, try to limit your added sugars to 6 teaspoons a day if you eat about 1,600 calories, 12 teaspoons at 2,200 calories, or 18 teaspoons at 2,800 calories. These amounts are intended to be averages over time. The patterns are illustrations of healthful proportions in the diet, not rigid prescriptions.

Added sugars are in foods like candy and soft drinks, as well as jams, jellies, and sugars you add at the table. Some added sugars are also in foods from the food groups, such as fruit canned in heavy syrup and chocolate milk. The chart on page 16 shows the approximate amount of sugars in some popular foods.

Salt and Sodium

Do I have to give up salt?

No. But most people eat more than they need. Some health authorities say that sodium intake should not be more than 2,400 mg. Nutrition labels also list a Daily Value (upper limit) of 2,400 mg per day for sodium. Much of the sodium in people's diets comes from salt they add while cooking and at the table. (One teaspoon of salt provides about 2,000 mg of sodium.)

Go easy on salt and foods that are high in sodium, including cured meats, luncheon meats, and many cheeses, most canned soups and vegetables, and soy sauce. Look for lower salt and no-salt-added versions of these products at your supermarket.

The amount of sodium in different types of foods should be calculated wisely. Information on food labels can also help you make food choices to keep sodium moderate.

Where's The Salt?

Food Groups	Sodium, mg
Bread, Cereal, Rice, and Pasta	
Cooked cereal, rice, pasta, unsalted, 1/2cup	Trace
Ready-to-eat cereal, 1 oz.	100-360
Bread, 1 slice	110-175
Popcorn, salted, 1 oz.	100-420
Pretzels, salted, 1 oz.	130-880
Vegetable	
Vegetables, fresh or frozen, cooked without salt, 1/2 cup	Less than 70
Vegetables, canned or frozen with sauce, 1/2 cup	140-460
Tomato juice, canned, 3/4 cup	660
Vegetable soup, canned, 1 cup	820
Fruit	
Fruit, fresh, frozen, canned, 1/2 cup	Trace
Milk, Yoghurt, and Cheese	
Milk, 1 cup	120
Yogurt, 8 oz.	160
Natural cheeses, 1-1/2 oz.	110-450
Process cheeses, 2 oz.	800
Meat, Poultry, Fish, Dry Beans, Eggs, and Nuts	
Fresh meat, poultry, fish, 3 oz.	Less than 90
Tuna, canned, water pack, 3 oz.	300
Bologna, 2 oz.	580
Ham, lean, roasted, 3 oz.	1,020
Peanuts, roasted in oil, salted, 1 oz.	120

Food Groups	Sodium, mg
Other	
Salad dressing, 1 tbsp.	75-220
Ketchup, mustard, steak sauce, 1 tbsp.	130-230
Soy sauce, 1 tbsp.	1,030
Salt, 1 tsp.	2,325
Dill pickle, 1 medium	930

Breads, Cereals, Rice, and Pasta

Why are breads, cereals, rice, and pasta important?

These foods provide complex carbohydrates (starches), which are an important source of energy, especially in low-fat diets. They also provide vitamins, minerals, and fibre. The Food Guide Pyramid suggests 6 to 11 servings of these foods a day.

What counts as a serving?

- 1 slice of bread
- 1 ounce of ready-to-eat cereal
- 1/2 cup of cooked cereal, rice, or pasta

Aren't starchy foods fattening?

No. It's what you add to these foods or cook with them that adds most of the calories. For example: margarine or butter on bread, cream or cheese sauces on pasta, and the sugar and fat used with the flour in making cookies.

Here are some selection tips:

- To get the fiber you need, choose several servings a day of foods made from whole grains, such as whole-wheat bread and whole-grain cereals.

- Choose most often foods that are made with little fat or sugars. These include bread, english muffins, rice, and pasta.
- Baked goods made from flour, such as cakes, cookies, croissants, and pastries, count as part of this food group, but they are high in fat and sugars.
- Go easy on the fat and sugars you add as spreads, seasonings, or toppings.
- When preparing pasta, stuffing, and sauce from packaged mixes, use only half the butter or margarine suggested; if milk or cream is called for, use lowfat milk.

Vegetables

Why are vegetables important?

Vegetables provide vitamins, such as vitamins A and C, and folate, and minerals, such as iron and magnesium. They are naturally low in fat and also provide fibre. The Food Guide Pyramid suggests 3 to 5 servings of these foods a day.

What counts as a serving?

- 1 cup of raw leafy vegetables
- 1/2 cup of other vegetables, cooked or chopped raw
- 3/4 cup of vegetable juice

Here are some selection tips:

- Different types of vegetables provide different nutrients. For variety eat:
    - dark-green leafy vegetables (spinach, romaine lettuce, broccoli);
    - deep-yellow vegetables (carrots, sweet potatoes);
    - starchy vegetables (potatoes, corn, peas);

- legumes (navy, pinto, and kidney beans, chickpeas);
- other vegetables (lettuce, tomatoes, onions, green beans).

☞ Include dark-green leafy vegetables and legumes several times a week—they are especially good sources of vitamins and minerals. Legumes also provide protein and can be used in place of meat.

☞ Go easy on the fat you add to vegetables at the table or during cooking. Added spreads or toppings, such as butter, mayonnaise, and salad dressing, count as fat.

☞ Use low-fat salad dressing.

Fruits

Why are fruits important?

Fruits and fruit juices provide important amounts of vitamins A and C and potassium. They are low in fat and sodium. The Food Guide Pyramid suggests 2 to 4 servings of fruits a day.

What counts as a serving?

☞ a medium apple, banana, or orange

☞ 1/2 cup of chopped, cooked, or canned fruit

☞ 3/4 cup of fruit juice

Here are some selection tips:

☞ Choose fresh fruits, fruit juices, and frozen, canned, or dried fruit. Pass up fruit canned or frozen in heavy syrups and sweetened fruit juices unless you have calories to spare.

☞ Eat whole fruits often—they are higher in fibre than fruit juices.

☞ Have citrus fruits, melons, and berries regularly. They are rich in vitamin C.

- ☞ Count only 100 percent fruit juice as fruit. Punches, ades, and most fruit "drinks" contain only a little juice and lots of added sugars. Grape and orange sodas don't count as fruit juice.

Meat, Poultry, Fish, Dry Beans, Eggs, and Nuts

Why are meat, poultry, fish, and other foods in this group important?

Meat, poultry, and fish supply protein, B vitamins, iron, and zinc. The other foods in this group — dry beans, eggs, and nuts — are similar to meats in providing protein and most vitamins and minerals. The Food Guide Pyramid suggests 2 to 3 servings each day of foods from this group. The total amount of these servings should be the equivalent of 5 to 7 ounces of cooked lean meat, poultry, or fish per day.

What counts as a serving?

- ☞ Count 2-3 ounces of cooked lean meat, poultry, or fish as a serving. A 3-ounce piece of meat is about the size of an average hamburger, or the amount of meat on a medium chicken breast half.
- ☞ For other foods in this group, count 1/2 cup of cooked dry beans or 1 egg as 1 ounce of lean meat. 2 tablespoons of peanut butter or 1/3 cup of nuts count as 1 ounce of meat (about 1/3 serving).

Counting to see if you have an equivalent of 5-7 ounces of cooked lean meat a day is tricky. Portion sizes vary with the type of food and meal. For example, 6 ounces might come from:

- 1 egg (count as 1 oz. of lean meat) for breakfast;
- 2 oz. of sliced turkey in a sandwich at lunch; and
- a 3 oz. cooked lean hamburger for dinner.

Lean Choices

Beef
Roasts/Steaks: *Round, Loin, Sirloin, Chuck Arm*

Pork
Roasts/Chops: *Tenderloin, Center Loin, Ham*

Veal
All cuts except ground

Lamb
Roasts/Chops: *Leg, Loin, Fore Shanks*

Chicken & Turkey
Light & dark meat, without the skin

Fish & Shellfish
Most are low in fat; those marinated or canned in oil are higher

Here are some selection tips:

☞ Choose lean meat, poultry without skin, fish, and dry beans and peas often. They are the choices lowest in fat.

☞ Prepare meats in low-fat ways:

- Trim away all the fat you can see.
- Broil, roast, or boil these foods, instead of frying them.

☞ Go easy on egg yolks; they are high in cholesterol. Use only one yolk per person in egg dishes. Make larger portions by adding extra egg whites.

☞ Nuts and seeds are high in fat, so eat them in moderation.

Milk, Yogurt, and Cheese

Why are milk products important?

Milk products provide protein, vitamins, and minerals. Milk, yogurt, and cheese are the best source of calcium. The Food

Guide Pyramid suggests 2 to 3 servings of milk, yogurt, and cheese a day—2 for most people, and 3 for women who are pregnant or breastfeeding, teenagers, and young adults to age 24.

What counts as a serving?

☞ 1 cup of milk or yogurt

☞ 1-1/2 ounces of natural cheese

☞ 2 ounces of process cheese

Here are some selection tips:

☞ Choose skim milk and non-fat yogurt often. They are lowest in fat.

☞ 1-1/2 to 2 ounces of cheese and 8 ounces of yogurt count as a serving from this group because they supply the same amount of calcium as 1 cup of milk.

☞ Cottage cheese is lower in calcium than most cheeses. One cup of cottage cheese counts as only 1/2 serving of milk.

☞ Go easy on high fat cheese and ice cream. They can add a lot of fat (especially saturated fat) to your diet.

☞ Choose "part skim" or lowfat cheeses when available and lower fat milk desserts, like ice milk or frozen yogurt.

The Pyramid Food Choices Chart

The following chart lists commonly used foods in each food group and the amount of fat in each. Only a few of the thousands of foods we eat are listed. However, they will give you an idea of foods from each food group that are higher and lower in fat.

The Food Guide Pyramid symbol (▼) next to the food item means that food is one of the lowest fat choices you can make in that food group.

You can use the food label to count fat in specific foods. Many labels on foods list the grams of fat in a serving.

How much is a gram of fat?

To help you visualize how much fat is in these foods, keep in mind that 1 teaspoon (1 pat) of butter or margarine has 4 grams of fat.

Amount of Food	Servings	Grams of Fat
Bread, Cereal, Rice, and Pasta Group		
Eat 6 to 11 servings daily		
Bread, 1 slice	**1**	**1**
Hamburger roll, bagel, english muffin, 1	**2**	**2**
Tortilla, 1	**1**	**3**
Rice, pasta, cooked, 1/2 cup	**1**	**Trace**
Plain crackers, small, 3-4	**1**	**3**
Breakfast cereal, 1 oz.	**1**	*
Pancakes, 4" diameter, 2	**2**	**3**
Croissant, 1 large (2 oz.)	**2**	**12**
Doughnut, 1 medium (2 oz.)	**2**	**11**
Danish, 1 medium (2 oz.)	**2**	**13**
Cake, frosted, 1/16 average	**1**	**13**
Cookies, 2 medium	**1**	**4**
Pie, fruit, 2-crust, 1/6 8" pie	**2**	**19**
* Check product label		
Vegetable Group		
Eat 3 to 5 servings daily		
Vegetables, cooked, 1/2 cup	**1**	**Trace**

Amount of Food	Servings	Grams of Fat
Vegetables, leafy, raw, 1 cup	**1**	**Trace**
Vegetables, non-leafy, raw, chopped, 1/2 cup	**1**	**Trace**
Potatoes, scalloped, 1/2 cup	**1**	**4**
Potato salad, 1/2 cup	**1**	**8**
French fries, 10	**1**	**8**
Fruit Group		
Eat 2 to 4 servings daily		
Whole fruit: medium apple, orange, banana	**1**	**Trace**
Fruit, raw or canned, 1/2 cup	**1**	**Trace**
Fruit juice, unsweetened, 3/4 cup	**1**	**Trace**
Avocado, 1/4 whole	**1**	**9**
Milk, Yogurt, and Cheese Group		
Eat 2 to 3 servings daily		
Skim milk, 1 cup	**1**	**Trace**
Nonfat yogurt, plain, 8 oz.	**1**	**Trace**
Lowfat milk, 2 percent, 1 cup	**1**	**5**
Whole milk, 1 cup	**1**	**8**
Chocolate milk, 2 percent,1 cup	**1**	**5**
Lowfat yogurt, plain, 8 oz.	**1**	**4**
Lowfat yogurt, fruit, 8 oz.	**1**	**3**
Natural cheddar cheese, 1-1/2 oz.	**1**	**14**
Process cheese, 2 oz.	**1**	**18**
Mozzarella, part skim, 1-1/2 oz.	**1**	**7**
Ricotta, part skim, 1/2 cup	**1**	**10**

Amount of Food	Servings	Grams of Fat
Cottage cheese, 4 percent fat, 1/2 cup	**1/4**	**5**
Ice cream, 1/2 cup	**1/3**	**7**
Ice milk, 1/2 cup	**1/3**	**3**
Frozen yogurt, 1/2 cup	**1/2**	**2**
Meat, Poultry, Fish, Dry Beans, Eggs, and Nuts Group		
Eat 5 to 7 oz. daily		
Lean meat, poultry, fish, cooked	**3 oz***	**6**
Ground beef, lean, cooked	**3 oz***	**16**
Chicken, with skin, fried	**3 oz***	**13**
Bologna, 2 slices	**1 oz***	**16**
Egg, 1	**1 oz***	**5**
Dry beans and peas, cooked, 1/2 cup	**1 oz***	**Trace**
Peanut butter, 2 tbsp.	**1 oz***	**16**
Nuts, 1/3 cup	**1 oz***	**22**
* Ounces of meat these items count as		
Fats, Oils, and Sweets		
Use sparingly		
Butter, margarine, 1 tsp.	-	**4**
Mayonnaise, 1 tbsp.	-	**11**
Salad dressing, 1 tbsp.	-	**7**
Reduced calorie salad dressing, 1 tbsp.	-	*
Sour cream, 2 tbsp.	-	**6**
Cream cheese, 1 oz.	-	**10**
Sugar, jam, jelly, 1 tsp.	-	**0**
Cola, 12 fl. oz.	-	**0**
Fruit drink, ade, 12 fl. oz.	-	**0**

Amount of Food	Servings	Grams of Fat
Chocolate bar, 1 oz.	-	**9**
Sherbet, 1/2 cup	-	**2**
Fruit sorbet, 1/2 cup	-	**0**
Gelatin dessert, 1/2 cup	-	**0**
* Check product label		

What about alcoholic beverages?

If adults choose to drink, they should have no more than 1 to 2 drinks a day. Alcoholic beverages provide calories, but little or no nutrients. These standard-size drinks each provide about the same amount of alcohol.

Alcoholic Beverages	Calories
Beer, 12 fl. oz. (1 regular can)	**150**
Wine, dry, 5 fl. oz.	**100**
Liquor, 1-1/2 oz.*	**100**
* A mixer such as a soft drink will add more calories	

How To Rate Your Diet

You may want to rate your diet for a few days. Follow these four steps.

Step 1

Jot down everything you ate yesterday for meals and snacks.

	Grams of Fat
Total	

Step 2

Write down the number of grams of fat in each food you list.

- ☞ Use the Pyramid Food Choices Chart to get an idea of the number of grams of fat to count for the foods you ate.
- ☞ Use nutrition labels on packaged foods you ate to find out the grams of fat they contained.

Step 3

Answer these questions:

- ☞ Did you have the number of servings from the five major food groups that are right for you? (See page 144 to determine the number of servings that are right for you.)

	Circle the Servings Right for You	Servings You Had
Grain Group Servings	**6 7 8 9 10 11**	
Vegetable Group Servings	**3 4 5**	
Fruit Group Servings	**2 3 4**	
Milk Group Servings	**2 3**	
Meat Group (ounces)	**5 6 7**	

How did you do? Not enough? About right?

- ☞ Add up your grams of fat listed in Step 2. Did you have more fat than the amount right for you? (See table on pages 145-46.)

	Grams Right for You	Grams You Had
Fat	**53 73 93**	

How did you do? Too much? About right?

- ☞ Do you need to watch the amount of added sugars you eat? See the table on pages 152-53 to estimate the number of teaspoons of added sugars in your food choices.

	Teaspoons Right for You	Teaspoons You Had
Sugars	**6 12 18**	

How did you do? Too much? About right?

Step 4

Decide what changes you can make for a healthier diet. Start by making small changes, like switching to low-fat salad dressings or adding an extra serving of vegetables. Make additional changes gradually until healthy eating becomes a habit.

11
Therapeutic Diet

There are special dietary needs for some of the diseased, hence, proper balanced diet should be planned for such patients. Ahead is a suggestive table.

Health Disorder	Dietary Modification	Rationale or Comments
AIDS	Based on specific symptoms.	See Diarrhea and COPD
Anemia, folate deficiency	Recommend folic acid (folate) supplements. Increase dietary intake of dark-green, leafy vegetables.	Lab reports "megaloblastic" RBCs. Folate is essential for RBC production and maturation. Maternal deficiency prior to conception is associated with fetal neural tube defects (spina bifida).
Anemia, iron deficiency (called milk anemia in child who drinks excessive amounts of milk rather than eating iron-rich foods)	Give iron supplements and iron-rich diet that includes liver, red meats, whole grains, dark-green leafy vegetables, and cereals. Ensure adequate intake of vitamin C.	Lab reports "hypochromic" and "microcytic" RBCs. Milk and antacids impair absorption of iron supplements. Vit. C facilitates absorption of iron.
Anemia, pernicious	Administer B12.	Lab reports "megaloblastic" RBCs. Anemia is caused by malabsorption of B12.

Health Disorder	Dietary Modification	Rationale or Comments
Anemia, sickle cell	Increase fluids to at least 1½ times usual requirement for weight and age. Folic acid (folate) may be given.	Sickled cells tend to clump together, causing vaso- occlusion. Increased fluid intake results in hemodilution, which impedes the clumping process. Folic acid essential for normal RBC formation.
Arthritis	Maintain ideal body weight by limiting fat and caloric intake.	Excess weight causes stress on joints.
Burns	High kilocaloric and protein intake. Give vitamin and mineral supplements. Enteral or parenteral feedings if PO feedings inadequate.	Calories and protein needed for healing. Decreased level of consciousness, poor appetite, or paralytic ileus may interfere with PO intake.
Calculi, renal	Generous fluid intake. Dietary calcium adequate to maintain serum calcium and prevent excessive bone loss of calcium.	Calculi most often composed of calcium, which is more soluble in acidic urine. Dilute urine less likely to support stone formation.

Health Disorder	Dietary Modification	Rationale or Comments
Cancer	Varies according to site and type of cancer. Generally, increase calories and protein with low to moderate fat. When chemotherapy destroys taste buds, slightly salty or sour tastes are usually accepted best.	Progressive disease causes hypermetabolism, weight loss, negative nitrogen balance, and the use of fat and muscle tissue for energy.
Cardiovascular disease	Prudent diet: Control calories in accordance with ideal body weight. Diet to consist of: carbohydrate (mainly complex) = 50% of daily calories, protein = 20% of daily calories, and fat (mostly vegetable) = 30% of daily calories. Salt added lightly during cooking, but not at table. Avoid salty-tasting foods.	These are recommendations of the American Heart Association for prevention and treatment of CV disease. Fat has 9 cal/g, whereas protein and carbohydrates have 4 cal/g. Excess salt may cause edems, which may result in elevated B

Health Disorder	Dietary Modification	Rationale or Comments
Celiac disease	Exclude wheat, oats, rye, barley, and buckwheat products. Give potato, corn, and rice products.	Foods on "excluded list" cause diarrhea and GI villi atrophy in persons with this inborn disorder.
Cholecystitis or cholelithiasis	Low-fat or possibly a fat- free diet for a limited time.	Fat in duodenum stimulates gallbladder contraction, thereby causing pain. Fat-free diet for more than 1 month may result in essential fatty acid deficiency.
Cirrhosis	Increase calories. Protein as tolerated (usually limited). Moderate fat. Low sodium. MCT oil if fat poorly tolerated. BCAAs (branched-chain amino acids) may be used to provide protein.	Anorexia usually present. Low sodium does not eliminate edema but may slow its progression. BCAAs are amino acids that do not require metabolism by liver. Monitor serum ammonia level to assess dietary protein tolerance.

Health Disorder	Dietary Modification	Rationale or Comments
Constipation	Increase fluid and fibre intake. If enteral feedings are in use, try formula with added fiber. If fiber-containing formula is ineffective, try one that is fiber free. Corn syrup may be added to infant formula.	Extra fluids and fibere increase peristalsis. (High-fiber intake can result in constipation if fluid intake is inadequate.) Corn syrup increases osmolarity of intestinal contents, thereby pulling water into gut and softening stool.
COPD	Increase fats. Decrease carbohydrates. Adequate fluids.	Fat has lower R/Q (respiratory quotient), uses less oxygen, and releases less CO_2than carbohydrates or protein. Fluids help liquefy pulmonary secretions.
Crohn's disease (regional enteritis)	Inactive periods: Regular diet with lactose and fiber limited. Exacerbations: Increase calories and protein. Parenteral (IV) feedings may be used.	Lactose poorly tolerated because of deficiency or absence of enzyme (lactase) needed for its digestion. Fiber is irritating to intestinal mucosa. Increased calories and protein needed because of fecal losses and malabsorption. Parenteral feeding allows gut to rest and heal.

Health Disorder	Dietary Modification	Rationale or Comments
Cystic fibrosis	Increase calories and protein. Fats as tolerated (decrease if stools are fatty). Encourage salty foods.	Genetic condition results in malabsorption of nutrients because of lack of adequate pancreatic enzymes and thick intestinal secretions. Excessive electrolytes are lost in sweat.
Decubitus (pressure ulcers)	Adequate kilocalories, protein, vitamin C, iron, and zinc.	These are critical components of the healing process.
Diabetes mellitus		
Type 1	Balance available glucose from food with available insulin. Exchange system often used. Dietary fiber may reduce rate of GI glucose absorption. For children, limitation of concentrated sweets may be only modification. Diet adjusted for individual life style and eating habits.	Pancreas produces limited or no insulin. Children have unpredictable activity spurts and high levels of growth hormone, causing blood glucose levels to be inconsistent even when a strict diet is followed. It is psychologically important for children to have diets similar to their peers.

Health Disorder	Dietary Modification	Rationale or Comments
Type 2	Primarily weight reduction and control of diet.	Reducing one's weight (if overweight) decreases insulin requirement.
MODY (mature-onset diabetes of the young)	Similar to Type 2 that occurs in adults.	
Diarrhoea	First, give diet of clear liquids (including ORS [oral rehydration solutions]). NPO if PO intake causes increased stooling. Advance to full liquids if tolerated, then to BRAT diet (bananas, rice, applesauce, and tea or toast).	ORS contain fluids and electrolytes. Elements of BRAT diet contain pectin and nonirritating carbohydrates.
Diverticulitis	High fibre during remissions. Bland diet during exacerbations. Elemental formulas or parenteral feedings may be used.	High fibre helps to promote peristalsis and may prevent material from remaining in diverticula but is not tolerated during exacerbations. Elemental formulas (predigested) or parenteral feedings allow gut to rest.

Health Disorder	Dietary Modification	Rationale or Comments
Dumping syndrome	Alternate liquids and dry foods. Avoid simple carbohydrates such as fruit juices or sodas. Dilute concentrated tube-feeding formulas.	Alternation of liquid and dry foods puts less food in solution, thereby decreasing osmolarity of gut contents. Simple carbohydrates trigger rapid release of insulin, resulting in hypoglycemia after the GI supply of glucose diminishes. Concentrated tube-feeding formulas attract water to the gut.
Edema	Control sodium. Provide adequate protein.	Edema may be caused by excess sodium or decreased albumin levels, or both.
Esophagitis	Give small, frequent meals. Promote weight loss if overweight. Avoid caffeine, pepper, and any food not well tolerated. Chew food thoroughly. Avoid lying down after meals.	Large meals, obesity, or lying down causes increased abdominal pressure resulting in esophageal reflux. Foods avoided are those that cause irritation. Hiatal hernia often results in esophagitis.

Health Disorder	Dietary Modification	Rationale or Comments
Fracture	Adequate protein, calcium, phosphorus, and vitamins A, C, and D. Dairy products are excellent sources for the above nutrients except for vitamin C. Citrus fruits provide vitamin C.	Adequate protein and vitamin C needed for collagen formation. Adequate calcium and phosphorus needed for bone strength. Vitamins A and D necessary for bone cell development, protein synthesis, and mineralization.
Gallbladder disease	See Cholecystitis	
Gastroesophageal reflux disorder (GERD)	Avoid chocolate, fatty foods, peppermint and spearmint oils, caffeine, and alcohol. Encourage protein-rich foods.	Listed foods lower (loosen) esophageal sphincter pressure, which results in reflux. Protein increases (tightens) sphincter pressure.
Gout	Encourage fluids. Limit fats. Decrease high-purine foods such as meats (especially organ meats), fish, fowl, lentils, whole grains, asparagus, mushrooms, spinach, cauliflower, and alcohol.	Extra fluid promotes uric acid excretion and helps prevent renal stone formation. Fats prevent excretion of uric acid. Purine breaks down to form uric acid.

Health Disorder	Dietary Modification	Rationale or Comments
Hepatic encephalopathy	Limit protein intake. Essential amino acids may be used (given IV).	On the limited-protein diet, essential amino acids receive top priority because they cannot be manufactured by the body. Ammonia improperly removed from serum by liver causes abnormal CNS symptoms. See Cirrhosis.
Hepatitis	High calorie and protein. Moderate fat. Avoid alcohol.	Anorexia is major problem. Moderation of fat promotes liver regeneration and healing. Alcohol is detoxified by the liver.
Hiatal hernia	Same indications as Esophagitis.	
Hypertension	Control calories to avoid excess weight. Limit sodium. Increase foods high in potassium (fruits and vegetables) and calcium (low-fat dairy products). DASH diet	Obesity increases risk of hypertension. Although the role of sodium in hypertension is debated, research shows that limiting dietary sodium and increasing potassium and calcium can lower blood pressure.

Health Disorder	Dietary Modification	Rationale or Comments
Irritable bowel syndrome	Regular diet when asymptomatic. Bland diet during exacerbation.	Bland diet decreases GI irritation.
Lactose intolerance	Reduce lactose (milk sugar) intake.	Condition may be partial or complete and may be inherited or due to stress or GI irritation.
Nausea/vomiting	Clear liquids. Offer ORS every 20–30 min.	Clear liquids prevent dehydration. ORS replaces electrolytes lost in emesis.
Nephrosis or nephrotic syndrome	Increase protein in diet unless accompanied by renal failure or elevated BUN. No salt added at table.	Protein is lost in urine in this disorder. Salt restriction does not remove edema but may limit its increase.
Obesity	Decrease calories. Modify food habits.	One pound of adipose (fat) tissue is roughly equivalent to 3500 Kcal. An increase or decrease of 500 Kcal a day leads to 1 lb weight gain or loss per week.

Health Disorder	Dietary Modification	Rationale or Comments
Osteoporosis	Ensure adequate dietary calcium by consuming dairy products or by taking supplemental calcium. Encourage exercise as tolerated.	Adequate dietary calcium and adequate exercise thought to be preventive.
Ostomy	Progress from clear liquid to low-residue, high-calorie diet. Maintain until desirable weight attained. Gradually add fibre (individual tolerance varies), avoiding gas- forming foods (based on individual tolerance). Ileal resections make B12injections necessary.	Ostomies result in increased nutrient losses (including electrolyte) from GI tract. Diet is individualized to avoid foods that cause patient to have excess stooling or gas. Intrinsic factor not available following ileal resection; therefore, B12cannot be absorbed through GI tract.
Pancreatitis	High protein, high carbohydrate with fat added to tolerance. Eliminate gastric stimulants such as coffee, tea, alcohol, and pepper. Withhold oral feedings during exacerbations.	Tolerance of fat is judged by fat in stools, abdominal distention, or abdominal discomfort. Gastric stimulants cause irritating pancreatic enzymes to be secreted.

Health Disorder	Dietary Modification	Rationale or Comments
Peptic ulcer	Bland diet with small, frequent feedings if ulcer is active. Avoid meat extract, pepper, caffeine, and alcohol.	Meat extracts stimulate stomach acid secretion. Obvious irritating foods avoided.
Phenylketonuria	Control phenylalanine (an essential amino acid) in diet. Breast-feeding is contraindicated.	An inborn error results in a lack of enzyme needed to catabolize phenylalanine.
Renal dialysis	Generous calories. Supplement of water- soluble vitamins. Limit fluids, protein, potassium, sodium, and phosphates.	See Renal Failure.
Renal failure, acute	Restrict protein until BUN and serum creatinine are normal. Restrict fluids during oliguric phase. Replace electrolyte deficits. (Avoid giving potassium during oliguric phase.)	Urea (BUN) and creatinine are the end products of protein metabolism. If kidneys are unable to remove urea, blood levels rise and affect CNS. Serum potassium levels may fluctuate rapidly.

Health Disorder	Dietary Modification	Rationale or Comments
Renal failure, chronic	Restrict protein proportionate to kidney function. Prevent weight loss by including sufficient calories. Amino acids may be given. Restrict potassium and phosphate intake.	Urea and creatinine accumulate in blood from protein breakdown. Addition of essential amino acids may be indicated if protein tolerance is less than 20 g/24 h. (Monitor BUN and creatinine.) Diseased kidneys do not effectively remove potassium, phosphates, urea, or creatinine from the blood.
Surgery	Adequate protein, calories, iron, and vitamin C.	Listed nutrients are needed for connective tissue (collagen) formation.
Ulcerative colitis	Low-lactose and low- residue diet. (Avoid dairy products and residue, no alcohol, no fried foods, no raw or cooked whole vegetables.) Regular diet during remission.	Stressed mucosa results in impaired ability to produce lactase, which leads to lactose intolerance. Residue (any material that ends up as faecal mass) is irritating.

Bibliography

1. Diet & Nutrition: A Holistic Approach: Rudolph Ballentine, Himalayan Institute Press, 2007.

2. Food Matters: A Guide to Conscious Eating, Simon & Schuster, 2008.

3. Natural Healing Wisdom & Know How: Useful Practices, Recipes, and Formulas for a Lifetime of Health: Amy Rost, Black Dog & Leventhal Publishers.

4. The Green Pharmacy: U. Erasmus, Rodale Press, 1997.

5. Natural Medicines: Dr. Debasish Kundu and Dr. Malik A.K. Awan (Kruger Brentt, U.K.).

6. Complete Food and Nutrition Guide: Roberta Larson Duyff, American Dietetic Association, 2002.

7. Materia Medica for the New Age Man: Dr. Debasish Kundu (Originals).

Notes on Spagyrics

By Dr. Debasish Kundu

Rs. 395/- US $ 21.50 Paperback

In this book author briefly discusses the principles of Alchemy with some exceptional notes on Sexual and Spiritual Alchemy.

CONTENTS: Note to the Readers, Foreword, Preface, Introduction, History of Alchemy, Spagyrics, Principles of Spagyrics, The Quest for the Quintessence, Plant Alchemy, Energetic Spagyrics, The Three Philosophical Principles, Spagyric Electro-Homoeopathy, Energy in the Organism, Herbal Medicine, Spiritual Alchemy, Sexual Alchemy, Spagyric Meditation, Hermetic Philosophy, Fermentation and Distillation of Wine Spirit, Spagyric Experiments, Explanation of Some Spagyrics Terms, Bibliography

Materia Medica and Practice of Medicine in Electro-Homoeopathy

By Dr.Debasish Kundu

Rs. 395/- US $ 21.50 Paperback

CONTENTS: Foreword, Preface, Electrohomoeopathy-An Introduction, Life History of Count Cesare Mattei, Preparation of Electro Homoeopathic Remedies, Electrohomoeopathy Formulas, Constitution and Temperament, Materia Medica of Electrohomoeopathy Medicines, Examination of the Patient, General Rules for Using the Medicines, Practice of Medicine, Points for External Application, Chief Points and their Uses, Clinical Index, Bibliography

Treatise on Spagyric Homoeopathic Pharmacy

By Dr. Debasish Kundu & Dr. Vijay Kant Agnihotri, Sr. Scientist, CSIR, Forewarded By Prof. Raffaele Pezzani, University of Padova, Italy

Rs. 395/- US $ 21.50 Paperback

It features all necessary information about the method of preparations and formulations of Zimpel, Krauss and Bernus. It is the only book which has incorporated Spagyrics formulas of Zimpel brought back from the lost fragments of time.

According to Prof. Pezzani, it is definitely a valuable guide, a friend that every Electrohomeopathy (according to Mattei) practitioner should possess. It is a must have collection for everyone.

CONTENTS: Dedication, Foreword, Preface, Spagyric Homeopathic Pharmacy, Electrohomoeopathy Formulas, Spagyrics after Zimpel, Krauss and Bernus, Medicinal Plants, Tables of Essential Oil Yielding Plants, Bibliography

Materia Medica for the New Age Man

By Dr. Debasish Kundu, Dr A.Jayasuriya, Chancellor, The Open International University, Colombo and Edited by Dr. M Ahmed, Member, Bangladesh Homeopathy Board, Dhaka

Rs. 450/- US $ 24.50 Hardbound

This is the only book which covered all therapeutic schools of Homeopathy, from Gemmotherapy, Lithotherapy, Bach flower to Spagyric Homeopathy.

CONTENTS: Foreword to the Second Edition, Introduction, Introduction to Homeopathy, Evolution of Disease, Introduction to Vital Force, Miasms, Homeopathic Pharmacy, Case Taking, Doctrine of Dosage, Therapeutic Schools of Homeotherapeutics at a Glance, Nosodes and Sarcodes, Materia Medica, Clinical Index of Homeopathic Remedies, Mother Tinctures (External Use), Do's and Don'ts for Patients, Clinical Tips for Dummies, General Index of Remedies, References

Treatise on Electro-Homoeopathic Pharmacy

By Dr. Debasish Kundu & Dr.Ajit Singh, Foreworded By Prof. Fabio R Ambrosi, Chairman, Mattei Archieves, Italy

Rs. 195/- US $ 15.50 Paperback

CONTENTS: Foreword, Preface, Introduction to Electro Homoeopathic Pharmacy, Laboratory Equipments Used in Electro Homoeopathy Pharmacy, Vehicles used in Electrohomoeopathy, Sources of Electro Homoeopthic Medicines, Collection of Medicinal Plants, Cohobation: An Extraordinary Pharmacy, Methods of Preparation of Spagyric Medicines, Quality Control Procedures, Pharmacodynamics of Electrohomoeopathy Essences, Dosages and Mode of Administration, List of Medicinal Plants Used in

Electrohomoeopathic Remedies, Appendix 1: Terminology, Appendix 2: Prescription Writing, Appendix 3: Biographies, Appendix 4: Apparatus, Bibliography

Essentials of Acupuncture

By Dr. Debasish Kundu & Prof. Choo Led Sin, Chairman, International Federation of Acupuncture, Singapore

Rs. 995/- US $ 40.00 Hardbound

The Only Book which deals with Acupuncture Anaesthesia

CONTENTS: Preface, Introduction, History of Acupuncture, Philosophy of Acupuncture, Five Elements Theory, Diagnosis in Traditional Chinese Medicine, Evaluation and Diagnosis, The Concept of Qi, Management & Research on Some Disorders, How Acupuncture Works, Acupuncture Anesthesia, Laser Acupuncture, Auriculotherapy, Atlas of Acupuncture Points, Therapeutics of Common Ailments, Therapeutics of Common Ailments, Infertility, Impotence and Acupuncture, Acupuncture in Hairfall, Does Acupuncture Hurts, Related Therapies, Explanation of Some Terms, Marmapuncture, Bibliography

Cesare Mattei's Principles of Electro Homeopathy

Interpreted & Revised By Dr. Debasish Kundu

Rs. 395/- US $ 21.50 Paperback

The classic text has been Rewritten in simple language with much needed Interpretation & Revision. In some places the original French edition has been consulted, also enriched with footnotes wherever necessary.

CONTENTS: Preface by Editor, What is Electro-Homeopathy?, Names of the Electro-Homeopathic Remedies, General Information about the Electro-Homeopathic Remedies, Sphere of Action of the Remedies in Globules, General Remarks on the Electric Liquids, Their Mode of Application, Results of Experience, Doses and Method of Administration of the Remedies in Globules, Of Diagnosis, Principles and Rules for the Selection of the Appropriate Remedy, Easy Experiments for Beginners, Catalogue of Diseases Cured by Electro-Homeopathy, Appendix

Stepping Stones to Electo-Homoeopathy (Count Mattei's System of Medicine)

By A J L Gliddon(Original Edition with Vitiation of Blood and Lymph Theory)

Rs. 395/- US $ 21.50 Paperback

A brief insight into the discovery of electro homeopathy together with a rational explanation of the principles involved and the proposed medicines.

CONTENTS: Introduction , The Human Body, Count Mattei's Theories, Symptoms of Disease, The Electro-Homceopathic Remedies, The Globule Remedies, The Electricities, External Use of Electricities, External Use of Globules, Baths, Compresses, etc., How to Select the Remedies, How to Determine the Dose, Dilutions, Dry Globules, Table of Doses, Minute Doses, Effects of the Remedies, Other Hygienic Helps, Diet, Dress, Pure Air, etc.

Essentials of Trace Elements & Biochemic Medicine

By Prof. Dr. Debasish Kundu, Edited By Prof. Seyed Farzin Hassanzadeh Salehian Ph.D. (Iran)

Rs. 350/- US $ 19.00 Paperback

Cell Salts or Bioplasgens have always been considered an important part of healing in Homeopathy and Spagyrics. This book contains all essential materials concerning Trace Elements & Bioplasgen and their relationship with Spagyrics, Clinical Materia Medica with useful suggestions.

CONTENTS: Preface, Introduction to Trace Elements & Bioplasgens, The Functions of The Cell, Astrology and Bioplasgens, Minerals, Trace Elements, Materia Medica of the Bioplasgens, Bio-combinations, Bibliography

A Textbook on Food, Nutrition and Dietetics

By Dr. Debasish Kundu Editor Dr. Malik A.K. Awan Ph.D. (London), Associate Editor Prof. Seyed Farzin Hassanzadeh Salehian Ph.D.(Iran)

Rs. 495/- US $ 20.00 Paperback

CONTENTS: Preface, Relationship between Food, Nutrition & Health, History of Nutrition, Functions of Food, Digestion of Food, Food and Nutrition, Nutrition, Diet & Development, Nutrition & Diet Therapy, Nutrition for Infants, Children, Adults, Women and Elderly, Ideal Diet Plan, The Food Pyramid, Therapeutic Diet, Bibliography

Notes on MJT (Forensic Medicine & Toxicology)

By Dr. Debasish Kundu Ph.D. Assisted By Dr. Ravi Justin Raj NMD, LLB Edited By Dr. Malik A.K. Awan B.S., M.S. (Psychology), D.C.L., D.D. (U.S.A.), Ph.D. (London)

Rs. 550/- US $ 22.00 Paperback

CONTENTS: Part I: Forensic Medicine: Dedication , Preface , Introduction, Scope of Forensic Medicine, Aspects of Identification, Medico-legal Aspects of Death, Investigation of Death, Death by Asphyxia, Medico-legal Aspects of Injuries, Investigation of Wounds, Medico-legal Aspects of Sex Crimes, Medico-legal Aspects of Abortion, Forensic Pathology, Forensic Entomology, Radiation Poisoning, Medico-legal Sections in IPC, Cr PC, AND IE A, Part II: Toxicology: Introduction to Toxicology, General Approach to a Victim of Poison, Clinical Toxicology Laboratory, Practical Aspects of Analytical Toxicology, Toxicants of Public Health Hazard, Medical Toxicants, Environmental Toxicants, Abuse of Drugs, Natural Toxicants, Annexure I: Preparations of Reagents, Annexure II: Apparatuses, Annexure III: Glossary of Terms Used, Annexure IV: Abbreviations Used, Bibliography

Notes on Minor Surgery

By Dr. Debasish Kundu Ph.D. Guided & Edited by Dr. A.K. Banerjee M.B.B.S., M.D. (U.S.A.)

Rs. 395/- US $ 21.50 Paperback

CONTENTS: Part-I: Preface, Acharya Sushruta, Basic Surgical Procedures, Surgery of Some Common Conditions, Part II: Sterilisation, Suture Materials, Nomenclature of Operations, Planning for Operation, Anaesthesia,Operative Surgery, Postoperative Complications, Abscess Drainage, Venesection (Cut Down), Skin Grafting, Circumcision, Vasectomy, Hyderocele, Inguinal Hernia, Strangulated Inguinal Hernia, Femoral Hernia, Umbilical Hernia, Appendicetomy,

Abdominal Incisions, Peptic Ulcer, Vagotomy, Gastrojejumnostomy, Partial Gastrectomy, Closure of Perforated Peptic Ulcer, Right Hemicolectomy, Colostomy, Cholecystectomy, Choledocholithotomy (Supraduodenal), Spleenectomy, Lumbar Sympathectomy, Haemorrhoidectomy, Suprapubic Cystostomy, Prostatectomy, Exposure of Kidney , Exposure of the Ureter and Ureterolithotomy, Mastectomy, Thyroidectomy, Tracheostomy, Empyema Thoracis, Amputations, Bibliography

Principles and Practice of Naturopathy

By Dr. Debasish Kundu Editor Dr. Malik A. K. Awan Ph.D. (London) Associate Editor Prof. Sayed Farzin Hassanzadeh Salehian Ph.D.(Iran)

Rs. 750/- US $ 30.00 Paperback

CONTENTS: Foreword, Preface to the First Edition, Preface to the Third Edition, Naturopathy: Its Principles & Pioneers, Physiology, Food and Nutrition, Hygiene and Sanitation, Biology, Herbology, Medicinal Plants, Magnet Therapy, Yoga and Meditation, Massage Therapy, Medical Gymnastics, Chemistry, Bacteriology, Toxicology, Pathology, Osteology, Neurology, Ethics, Hydro Therapy and Helio Therapy, Colour Therapy, Fasting and Diet, Mud Therapy and Fango Therapy, Acupressure, Aromatherapy, Reflexology, Iridology, Vitamins and Balanced Diets, Bibliography

Diseases of Women (Adopted from Margaret Seifert's Krankheiten Der Franen)

By Dr. Shefalika Kundu, Edited By Dr. Debasish Kundu & Dr. Sudeshna Kundu

Rs. 350/- US $ 19.00 Paperback

The book is intended as a handbook on diseases of women with their Electrohomeopathic treatment. Besides an update on the literature on Contraception using Spagyrics , entirely new topics Anatomy of Uterus and Stages of development in Pregnancy are added.

CONTENTS: Preface to the Second Edition, Foreword to the First Edition, Preface, Introduction, Anatomy and Physiology of Sexual Organs of Women, General View of Treatment, Diseases and Their Treatment, Hygienic Care of the Body and Toilet, Anatomy of Uterus in Pregnancy, Notes on Various Diseases, Family Planning, Contraception in Electrohomoeopathy,Diet, Index of Diseases Discussed, Bibliography

Lectures on Materia Medica & Therapeutics

By Dr. H. D. Banerjee, Foreworded By M V Mattei, Thoroughly Revised & Edited By Prof. Dr. Debasish Kundu

Rs. 225/- US $ 18.00 Paperback

CONTENTS: Preface to the Third Edition, Preface to the Second Edition, Foreword to the First Edition, Introduction, On Electro-Homoeopathic Principles, On Principles of Orthodox School, On Homeopathic Principles , On Objections to Electro-Homoeopathy, Chemical Analysis of the Remedies, Dynamisation of the Remedies, On Minute Doses, On Frequency of the Doses, Purgatives in Electro-Homoeopathy, On Prescription Writing, Materia Medica & Therapeutics, On Therapeutics of the Remedies

Principles & Art of Cure in Electrohomeopathy

By Prof. Dr.Debasish Kundu Ph.D.

Rs. 195/- US $ 15.00 Paperback

CONTENTS: Introduction to Electrohomeopathy, Philosophy, The Discoverer, Principles of Nature, Introduction to Electrohomeopathy Medicines, The Iris science, Sources and preparation of Electrohomeopathy Medicines, Cohobation, Spagyric Tinctures, Classification of Electrohomeopathy Medicines, Classification, Preparation and Therapeutics uses of Electrohomeopathy Medicines, Potentisation of Electrohomeopathy Medicines and Electric fluids, Preparation and Therapeutic uses of Ointments and Lotions, Points for application Electric Fluids, Ointments and Lotions, Plain talks on using the medicines, Potentisation and Bio-Magnetism, The Similia of Electrohomeopathy, The Scientific basis of Electrohomeopathy System of Medicine, World's present day need of Electrohomeopathy, Clinical Index.

A Clinical Treatise on Cancer

By Prof. Dr.Debasish Kundu Ph.D. Forewarded By Dr. B.B. Upreti, Ph. D. General Secretary, All Nepal Electro-Homeo Medical Association, Hetauda, Nepal

Rs. 195/- US $ 15.00 Paperback

CONTENTS: Introduction, The Increase of Cancer and it's Causes, The Treatment of Cancer, Diet for Patients, Hygienic Care of the Patients

Books Published By LBO Publishing, 700 N Valley St., Suite B PMB 11884 Anaheim, CA 92801, USA Marketed In India Exclusively By Originals, Delhi

Pharmacodynamics in Spagyric Medicine(Plant Alchemy)

By Dr. Debasish Kundu & Dr.Sudeshna Kundu, Edited by Gisela Bruckel(Germany), El Akrem Hayouni (Tunisia), Forwarded by Dr.Peter Morrell (U.K.), Prof. Luigi Vernacchia & Dr.Fabio Ambrosi (Italy) Printed on Art Paper, USD ($) 70.00, Hardbound

It is the only trusted book to learn Sacred Alchemical Philosophy with Practical Laboratory Spagyrics, it covers from history & principles of Alchemy to the rarest topic Botanical Consciousness in Spagyrics, besides, Alchemy and the Zodiac Connection and how Spagyric Medicines work. In addition, detailed Pharmaceutical Process which are being carried out in most modern laboratories : from Apparatus, Vehicles, Sources of Medicines, Preparation of Spagyric Essences, quality control like Phytochemical Analysis, etc. , all major Spagyric Methods known to mankind, incl., Mattei, Zimpel, Junius, Solaris, Krauss,etc., besides the sacred Indian, Arabian and Chinese methods, Doctrine of Dosage, and much more. An Encyclopedia of Spagyrics or Plant Alchemy in one nutshell.

This work is edited by Gisela Bruckel, who is a Pharmacist and her Pharmacy in Wurzburg was the Main Dealer of Mattei Remedies in Europe till M V Mattei era, and Prof. El Akrem Hayouni, World famous authority on Plant Alchemy.

CONTENTS: Foreword, Preface, Part 1: Introduction to Spagyric Medicine, History of Alchemy, Principles of Spagyrics, The Simila of Alchemy, Difference Between Homoeopathy and Spagyric Homoeopathy, Botanical Consciousness in Spagyrics, Micronutrients and Spagyrics, Alchemy and the Zodiac Connection, How Spagyric Medicines Work, Alchemy and Spagyrics, Spagyrics : The Future in Medicine, Part 2: Pharmacy in Plant Alchemy, Pharmaceutical Process, Laboratory Apparatus, Vehicles Used in Plant Alchemy, Sources of Medicines, Preparation of Spagyric Essence, Spagyric Essence by Cohobation Method, Phytochemical Analysis of Plants, Different Spagyric Methods, Quality Control Procedures, Safety Measures in Laboratory, Doctrine of Dosage, Medicinal Plants, Terminology, Appendix, Bibliography

Mysticism, Romance & Secrets of Count Cesare Mattei (With Properly Transcripted Secret Formulas)

By Prof. Dr. Debasish Kundu , Ph.D. (U.S.A.)

Printed on Art Paper, USD ($) 40.00 Hard Bound

It is the Bible of Mattei Electrohomoeopathy : covering the true life of Cesare Mattei and properly transcripted Empirical Formulas & Secret Pharmacy of Electrohomoeopathy, incl. Medicinal Plants Used by Cesare Mattei.

Contributors-Prof. Raffaele Pezzani, University of Padova, Italy, Dr. Fabio R. Ambrosi, University of Sapienza, Rome, Italy, Prof. El Akrem Hayouni, University of Manouba, Tunisia, Allesandro Rapparini, Vice Pres., Archivio Museo Cesare Mattei, Bologna, Italy, Prof. Peter Morrell, Formerly Honorary Research Associate, History of Medicine, Staffordshire University, U.K., Dr. Terry Mitchell, Alchemist & Director, Phylak GmbH, U.K., Willow Morningsky, Spagyrist & Psychologist, Southern Oregon University, Ashland, Oregon, U.S.A. etc.

CONTENTS: Introduction, Dedication, Note to the Readers, Acknowledgements, Alchemist's Prayer, Preface, The Castle of Love, The Mystery Unveiled, Emerald Tablet of Cesare Mattei, Mysticism & Romance of Cesare Mattei, Electro Homoeopathy Pharmacology, Medicinal Plants Used by Cesare Mattei, Glossary of Pharmacological Terms, Bibliography

For Further Information and Ordering:
Originals/Low Price Publications
A-6, Second Floor, Nimri Commercial Centre,
Ashok Vihar Phase-4, Delhi - 110 052 (India)
Tel.: +91 11 2730 2453 Fax: 011 4706 1936
Mobile: 98100-12366
Website: www.Lppindia.com,
e-mail: info@Lppindia.com
info@Lbopub.com